T0181829

Occupational Health Ethics

Jacques Tamin

Occupational Health Ethics

From Theory to Practice

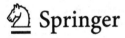 Springer

Jacques Tamin
Centre for Occupational
and Environmental Health
University of Manchester
Manchester, UK

ISBN 978-3-030-47285-6   ISBN 978-3-030-47283-2   (eBook)
https://doi.org/10.1007/978-3-030-47283-2

This Springer imprint is published by the registered company Springer Nature Switzerland AG
The registered company address is: Gewerbestrasse 11, 6330 Cham, Switzerland

This book is dedicated to the memory of my brother Sylvio (1959–2017) who practiced medicine and occupational health with the highest moral integrity, most ethical behavior and deepest compassion.

Acknowledgments

There are so many teachers and colleagues that have helped me on my journey as an OH professional and later as an ethicist that I could not possibly name them all. However, I am particularly grateful to Prof. Diana Kloss who taught me OH law and inspired me to find out more about law and ethics. I thank my Ph.D. supervisors Prof. Søren Holm and Dr. Sarah Devaney for their wise counsel and mentorship. I thank Prof. Raymond Agius for his support over many years and for being a beacon of integrity. There have been many outstanding OH professionals that I have had the privilege to work with, but I wish to express particular gratitude to members of the North West Audit Group (NWAG) and to Dorothy Howell and Joanne Carroll for the many hours we discussed difficult OH issues. I also wish to thank the book reviewers for their most helpful comments and feedback.

Prologue

I got to know Elsie (name changed to preserve anonymity) quite well in the last year of her life. I saw her in my occupational health clinics, during her brief periods of remission. She had battled metastatic cancer with courage and fortitude. She knew her prognosis was poor. She had been a ward clerk in the hospital for nearly 40 years. She was immensely proud of that service, and the small contribution (as she humbly saw it) she made to patient welfare. Her hope was to return to work once she was strong enough, and to end her working life "on a high note".

After endless courses of chemotherapy and radiotherapy, there was a time when she became well enough for us to plan a gradual return to work. She was overjoyed at the prospect, and so grateful for the chance of a final few months in the job she loved. She would soon be reaching retirement age but did not really want to retire.

I agreed on a "return to work" date with her manager, her general practitioner and treating specialists. I had planned a review shortly after her resumption. We planned to gradually increase her working hours, depending on how she coped with her residual fatigue. However, she failed to turn up for that review appointment, which was unusual. She *never* missed appointments. We tried to contact her, but her manager told us she had not attended work. We later received a call from a Human Resources (HR) manager to tell us she was no longer employed. She had had a deterioration a few days before she was due to resume. That had triggered the final stage of the HR attendance policy. He had visited her at home and terminated her employment!

I was distraught. I knew what this would have meant to her, especially that she would have felt such shame in being dismissed from work in this way. We finally managed to speak to her husband. He thanked us for our concern and our support during her illness. Elsie had died the day after she was sacked.

More than twenty years later, the memory of Elsie's pride in her contribution at work and the crushing blow of losing her job are still with me. Her story also reminds me that what we do, as occupational health professionals, matters in ways that are hard to quantify.

In a world where organizations place increasing emphasis on efficiency and productivity, values such as dignity and fairness may not feature highly. In the workplace, occupational health professionals have amongst their listed duties, "respecting human dignity" (ICOH 2014). I hope we always strive to respect the human dignity of those who can be at their most vulnerable. We may not always be successful, but we should not stop trying.

Contents

Contents

Abbreviations

AIDS	Acquired Immuno-Deficiency Syndrome
BMA	British Medical Association
BMJ	British Medical Journal
CA	Capability Approach
DOI	Digital Object Identifier
DPR	Doctor-Patient Relationship
EPP	Exposure-Prone Procedure
ERATOH	Ethics Reflection and Audit Tool in Occupational Health
ERATOM	Ethics Reflection and Audit Tool in Occupational Medicine
ESMPH	European Society for Philosophy of Medicine and Health Care
FFW	Fitness For Work
GDPR	General Data Protection Regulations
GMC	General Medical Council
GNP	Gross National Product
GP	General Practitioner
H&S	Health and Safety
HAVS	Hand-Arm Vibration Syndrome
HCW	Health Care Worker
HDI	Human Development Index
HIV	Human Immuno-deficiency Virus
HR	Human Resources
HSE	Health and Safety Executive
IC	Informed Consent
ICOH	International Commission on Occupational Health
IHR	Ill-Health Retirement
IRMP	Independent Registered Medical Practitioner
IT	Information Technology
MR	Management Referral
NHS	National Health Service
NWAG	North West Audit Group

OH	Occupational Health
OHP	Occupational Health Professional
OM	Occupational Medicine
PEP	Post-Exposure Prophylaxis
PH	Public Health
PTD	Permission To Disclose
RIDDOR	Reporting of Injuries, Disease and Dangerous Occurrences Regulations (UK)
UJIH-SC	Unemployment, Job Insecurity and Health Scientific Committee (of ICOH)
UK	United Kingdom
UN	United Nations
UNCRPD	UN Convention on the Rights of Persons with Disabilities
UNDP	United Nations Development Programme
US/USA	United States of America
WHO	World Health Organisation
WRFQ	Work Role Functioning Questionnaire
WRS	Work-Related Stress

Chapter 1
Introduction

This book is intended to be a practical ethics guide for practicing occupational health (OH) professionals. It is therefore primarily aimed at all those who practice OH in some way, whether as their main function, such as occupational physicians and occupational health nurses, or part-time, such as primary care physicians. OH is usually provided by a multi-disciplinary team nowadays, so I include other occupational health professionals (OHPs) such as physiotherapists, occupational therapists, occupational psychologists and technicians working in OH, in my target audience. It may also be of interest and relevance to others closely affiliated to OH services (and sometimes working within OH teams) such as occupational hygienists, occupational toxicologists and health and safety (H&S) professionals. I will use many examples from OH practice to discuss and reflect on the ethical issues, rather than use a didactic approach.

Although this book is not specifically aimed at employers, human resource (HR) professionals, trade union representatives, or employment lawyers, it may interest them to understand the ethical issues that their OH colleagues often grapple with, and the ways in which these challenges can be addressed and hopefully resolved.

Integrity

Before we look at ethical principles and theories to guide us through the OH moral maze, I would first like to mention the importance that I attach to personal and professional **integrity**. I have had the privilege of knowing and working with some OH professionals of the highest integrity. They would stand up for their beliefs and values in the most difficult and challenging of circumstances. I am in awe of them. I would like to believe that I also have acted and would always act with such integrity. At least, that is my hope. But I am not sure that I have always got it right. For those of you who also experience or have experienced such self-doubt, this book may be of special interest to you. It aims to help you reflect on the difficulties you face, and provide some guidance at what might be the best "moral" approach to that problem.

© Springer Nature Switzerland AG 2020
J. Tamin, *Occupational Health Ethics*,
https://doi.org/10.1007/978-3-030-47283-2_1

However, it seems pointless to me to seek the most morally correct solution unless we are prepared to act on it. Therein lies the crucial importance of moral courage and integrity.

The International Commission on Occupational Health (ICOH) also highlights the importance of integrity. It lists it as one of the three basic principles in its Code of Ethics. Of course, we are not alone in OH in needing to act with professional integrity. Health professionals in other disciplines can also be subjected to pressures, directly or indirectly, to act in ways which could be against a patient's best interest.

However, OH does have its special ethical challenges. The reasons for this will be explored in the next section.

Why OH Ethics?

In the preface to a previous edition of the UK Faculty of Occupational Medicine (FOM) guidance on ethics, Dr. David Snashall, then President of the FOM, stated:

> Practising occupational physicians probably think about ethics every day. At least they think about the subject more often than most doctors…

Why should practising occupational physicians think about ethics every day, or at least more often than most doctors? After all, they are not usually involved in life or death decisions, or complex moral issues around the beginning and end of life. Furthermore, the experience of thinking about ethics is not confined to the UK. For example, a study of OH physicians and nurses in Finland showed that 97% of them had experienced ethical issues in their OH practice. Nor does this concern only OH physicians and nurses: other members of a multidisciplinary OH team can be similarly affected.

So, what is it about OH that makes it so ethically problematic? Ethical difficulties that arise from OH practice may partly be explained by the *intrinsic* nature of the discipline of OH itself. The very fact that it places "dual obligations" (which will be explained in Chap. 2) on OH professionals produces a tension between their obligations to the two (or more) parties, especially when these obligations and/or the parties are in conflict. For example, a worker may believe himself to be too ill to work, whereas the employer does not believe this to be the case. Conversely, another worker may want to continue to work when his employer does not believe it to be safe for him to do so. Therefore, one can understand that on a day-to-day basis, OH professionals might give advice that one or other party might not like. Does this necessarily cause ethical problems? To understand where the ethical problems arise, it would be helpful to understand the basis of what might make one course of action morally preferable to another in our OH practice. We can gain such insights from our own personal moral values (within the context of our cultural and societal values); our professional training and development; an understanding of moral theories and approaches; and specific ethical codes or guidance written for OH professionals. The first section of this book deals with the theoretical underpinning of OH ethics by examining and applying moral theories and approaches in an OH context. But first, let us look at the role ethical codes play in guiding our practice.

Codes of Ethics

Although my aim is to generally keep references separate to the main text (mentioning them in the "Notes" section to each chapter instead), I believe that one cannot really discuss the topic of Codes of OH ethics without mentioning the seminal work of Peter Westerholm in this area. Most commentators who mention ethics codes in the OH context quote his work on this topic and I will do the same.

While Codes of ethics are generally useful and have an important role in guiding OH professionals on ethical issues, Westerholm nonetheless identifies three problem areas: "the interpretation problem, the multiplicity problem and the legislation problem." The difficulties in translating rules or guidance into real life situations, as well as contradictory advice within the codes, contribute to difficulties in *interpretation* of the codes. The number of different guidance and codes produced, some of which can be contradictory between each other, causes the *multiplicity* problem. The *legislation* problem arises when the question "what is the morally right thing to do?" is replaced by the narrower "what is legally permissible?". If codes are interpreted in this narrower way, then OH professionals might not develop through their reflective practice (which is a key professional behavior), instead they might blindly follow rules in an unthinking and minimalistic way.

At their best, they can be like a "lighthouse" (analogy by Westerholm 2009) shining light and guiding OH professionals through ethical uncertainties. In this regard, the example *par excellence* is the ICOH Code of Ethics. It defines and clarifies our moral priorities as OH professionals, and in so doing provides a bearing for our moral compass. Its importance is also highlighted by the fact that it is internationally recognized as being authoritative. However, it does not provide much detail (which is not necessarily a weakness), or much moral theory (which is not its intention in any case). On the other hand, it *does* articulate the "value set of OH professionals" (Westerholm 2009), and in so doing, acts as a "lighthouse" to guide us to practice OH ethically.

Scope of This Book

This book is written primarily for OH practitioners. I will mainly focus on the ethical issues that arise out of their OH practice. To that effect, I will choose the moral theories and approaches that I believe will best help us to discuss and reflect on these ethical concerns. However, as OH professionals we are also uniquely placed at the work-health interface. I believe that each of us has a chance to influence others (such as employers and rule-makers) to make the workplace a fairer, less discriminatory place, especially towards those who are more vulnerable. This then calls for an approach to arguing about social justice and fairness, so I will also consider the theoretical underpinning of such arguments (in Chap. 5).

But there are many areas that I will not consider in any great detail in this book. For example, I will briefly mention (in Chap. 9) what future OH may look like (and the corresponding ethical challenges they might bring), which include the impacts of globalization, demographic changes and newer technologies, but will not analyze the implications in depth. I think that these subjects could form the basis of a whole book by themselves! The other large topic I have not included in this book is the ethics of OH research (though I have mentioned a reference in the "Notes" section). I *do* consider research in OH to be something we should promote and foster. Indeed, evidence-based practice needs good research to have been conducted. The importance of evidence-based practice is highlighted at various points in this book. However, most OH professionals do not routinely carry out research, so this topic might have been of a more passing interest to them compared with the ethical difficulties they face in their everyday practice.

Moral Theories and Approaches

In this section, I will review the moral theories and approaches that will be used in the rest of book. Although the emphasis in this book is on "practical" OH ethics, we need to have sufficient understanding of moral theories which might underpin our ethical deliberations when confronted with these issues in the course of our practice. I will also briefly mention some of the theories or approaches that I will not be using.

The "Four Principles"

The "four principles" approach (often known as *principlism*), originally articulated by Beauchamp and Childress in 1979 is the cornerstone of biomedical and healthcare ethics. It was used for example in the Appleton consensus in 1989, when ethicists and physicians agreed on the ethical issues arising from patients deciding to forego medical treatment. Forty years on, the Beauchamp and Childress textbook of biomedical ethics has undergone many revisions and remains a classic. There are few students in the healthcare and associated professions, I would suggest, who would not be able to list the four principles, namely respect for autonomy, nonmaleficence, beneficence and justice. Let us now look at each of these in turn, in the context of the principles approach (as *per* Beauchamp and Childress).

Autonomy is defined as self-rule or self-governance, and at an individual level, this means one that is free from controlling interference by others and one has sufficient understanding to make a meaningful choice. *Respecting* a patient's autonomy, which is relevant to the healthcare and OH contexts, means that we "acknowledge their right to hold views, to make choices, and to take actions based on their values and beliefs". We will see later (in Chap. 3) how autonomy underpins the concept of "informed consent", with which we are familiar in both healthcare and OH practice. Indeed, autonomy is a key ethical principle, and in cases of ethical conflict, this often needs to be balanced against other competing ethical principles or values, to reach our "best" or preferred moral choice in that situation.

The principle of *nonmaleficence* is also one that resonates well with our values as healthcare professionals. We are used to the notion that first we must do no harm. However, this is one of the principles that can come into conflict with that of autonomy. If respecting the autonomy of one individual/patient/worker could lead to the harm of another or a group, which principle ought we give preference to? There are no easy answers to this. In the examples we will consider later (in Chaps. 6, 7 and 8), we will see that when we are balancing the autonomy of an individual against the possible harm to others, we need to evaluate the likelihood and the severity of that harm. That is, of course, a risk assessment process, which we will be very familiar with, as OH professionals.

Similarly, the principle of *beneficence* is one that we readily subscribe to as healthcare and OH professionals. Beauchamp and Childress make the point that contributing to others' (that is, patients') welfare is implicit in the healthcare context. I will later describe how our primary purpose, as OH professionals, is to protect the health of the worker (in Chap. 2), and so, our concern for the welfare of workers is a moral imperative for us. I see this as a positive, one of the "lighthouses" to illuminate our moral decision-making in OH. However, the principle of beneficence can also come into conflict with that of respect for autonomy, when a worker would rather choose a course that could put his life and health at risk. Ought we override this choice? If we do, we could be accused of acting *paternalistically*, which is generally not considered acceptable. I will illustrate the possible tension that can arise between the principles of beneficence and respect for autonomy in an OH context later in Chap. 7 ("Health surveillance").

The last of the "four principles" is *justice* (meaning fairness). In the healthcare context it is often used to mean *distributive* justice, that is, a fair and equitable sharing of resources that would help improve health and provide healthcare. In our OH context, we are mindful that there should not be unfair discrimination, for example, and justice can provide a conceptual underpinning for arguments in this area of ethics. As you will later see, I echo a plea made by others (in ICOH reports referred to in Chap. 5) that OH professionals should be active in helping the more **vulnerable** workers and individuals in our society. For that reason, I will cover some theories and concepts of justice (especially the *capability approach*) that I think are particularly relevant to OH, in Chap. 5.

In addition to the four principles, Beauchamp and Childress also specify four "rules", namely veracity, privacy, confidentiality and fidelity. These are relevant in our OH context, but I will not expand on the rules here. Instead, I will discuss fidelity in the context of our professional-worker relationship (Chap. 2), privacy and confidentiality in Chap. 4, and mention veracity in an ethical dilemma described in a case vignette (the case of Ernie) in Chap. 6.

Deontology

The best known of the moral theories that are based on duty, or deontology, is that of Kant. Those who criticize his approach point out, for example, its excessive formalism. However, some philosophers who favor this conceptual approach have shown how it can be applied to contemporary ethical debates. In any case, as healthcare and OH professionals, we are very comfortable with the idea that we have specific professional duties to patients, workers and others. These are usually specified by our regulators and in codes of ethics (see above), but I would suggest that through our education and training, many of these professional duties and attitudes become interwoven into the very fabric of who we are (in our professional roles). This approach gives us much guidance in what the morally right and professionally correct course of action should be. However, when different duties or obligations come into conflict, we still need to have a way of resolving such conflicts. For example, in OH practice, our main aim is to protect the health of workers. That is our primary duty. But what if this conflicts with our duty of confidentiality or our respect for a worker's autonomy? This could arise, for example, in health surveillance situations where a worker ought to be removed from exposure to a harmful agent to protect his health, but he disagrees with the OH professional and wishes to take the risk to his health. Such scenarios will be discussed in Chap. 7 ("Health surveillance").

Rights

We are probably all familiar with the notion of "human rights" and might think that the discourses from that perspective are a relatively recent phenomenon. However, philosophers from the seventeenth century have argued from a notion of entitlement to certain rights. This approach lost favor, when other schools of thought, such as utilitarianism, became prominent. There has been a resurgence of interest in human rights as a basis for political and moral debate globally, and this has been reflected in the UN's Universal Declaration of Human Rights in 1948. Further international endorsements have since given this declaration even greater currency. It has been the basis for the development of national and regional human rights legislation. Of particular interest to us in the world of work is Article 23, which not only iterates a right to work for everyone (think of the disabled, for instance), but also that this should be in *favorable conditions of work* (We will later see, in Chap. 5, that vulnerable workers are especially at risk of being in *unfavorable* working conditions). Another Article of special interest to us is Article 12, which specifies a right to privacy. I will be referring to a right to privacy in the context of informational privacy, in relation to confidentiality and disclosed information, in Chaps. 4 ("Confidentiality") and 6 ("Report writing").

Consequences

Another approach to moral theories is to see what the *consequences* would result from acting or not acting in a certain way, which action or inaction leads to the morally preferable or desired outcome. The best known of the consequentialist theories is the *utilitarian* approach. The latter approach is underpinned by the view that the morally correct approach is that which would maximize utility (such as happiness) for the greatest number. I will later touch on utilitarianism again in the context of theories of justice (in Chap. 5) but will not generally be using utilitarian arguments in our OH context. However, I will apply consequence-based arguments in some of the analyses of OH ethical problems. I think that looking at consequences may be fairly intuitive to those of us who face these problems at a practical level, rather than a purely theoretical one. For example, it may be reasonable to make a case that one should act in a certain way in a certain situation, based on our *duties*, but if the practical *consequence* of doing so results in bad outcomes (broadly conceived), then we may reject the duty-based argument. I am not suggesting that consequentialist arguments are always preferable, merely that we need to take account of several types of theories (and sometimes they may be in conflict) when we are faced with a practical ethical problem.

Summary

To summarize this section on the approach to moral theories that this book will take, I would say that it is a *pluralistic* approach that will be used. I will often use arguments derived from *principlism* in our OH situations, as much of OH is similar to healthcare, where the four principles are extensively used, so the approach works equally well in many OH situations. However, I will also use deontology-based, rights-based and consequentialist-based arguments where these approaches might help us understand an ethical issue better. To illustrate this, if we look at how we justify keeping worker information confidential, we can use duty-based (our fiduciary duty of confidentiality), rights-based (the worker's right to privacy) and consequence-based (worker trust in OH) as reasons why we should respect the confidentiality of that information (see Chap. 4). Throughout the book, I will make constant reference to our "dual obligations", which other healthcare professionals may not need to grapple with as much as we do, as OH practitioners. Furthermore, I will take our *primary duty to protect the health of workers* as a guide for our moral compass, to be the "lighthouse" in situations of ethical uncertainty (to paraphrase Westerholm).

Lastly, the above list is not intended to be a comprehensive summary of moral theories, it merely draws attention to those ethical theories and approaches I will mainly use in this book. There are many other moral theories that could be of interest to us, such as virtue theories and care theories, but I have not currently found an application for these in our OH context. I say *currently*, because moral theories continue to evolve, as does OH practice (as I will mention in Chap. 9). Indeed, I envisage that in future, more ethical theories will have direct appeal to OH ethical theory and practice. This is but the beginning.

A Guide for the Reader

This is an overview of how this book is structured.

The remaining chapters of this book are divided into two main parts. Part 1 (Chaps. 2–5) deals with the theoretical basis of OH ethics. In Part 2, I review some of the main OH practical activities through the lens of OH ethics (Chaps. 6–8), with Chap. 9 as the concluding chapter. Finally, the "notes" to each chapter, which include references and commentaries to provide supporting arguments and evidence for the contents of Parts 1 and 2, will be at the end of the book.

The following is a brief synopsis of each of the remaining chapters:

Chapter 2: The doctor-patient relationship and dual obligations in Occupational Health.

In this chapter, the similarities and differences between the OH professional-worker relationship and the "traditional" doctor-patient relationship are explored, particularly the role that *trust* plays in these relationships. The OH professional's duties to the worker and the employer (the "dual obligations") are reviewed and the ethical tensions that can arise from owing obligations to these parties are described. I suggest that an approach to reducing potential ethical conflicts would be to clarify our different OH *roles* in terms of the trust, power imbalance and fiduciary obligations that each role would entail. This would make it easier to explain to all parties which obligations take priority in different situations, and this transparency may help to improve trust in OH professionals.

Chapter 3: Consent.

This chapter on consent gives us an opportunity to consider one of the most important principles in healthcare ethics, namely **autonomy**. This is because our requirement to obtain patient or worker consent before we carry out any intervention is understood to reflect our respect for their autonomy. However, the wishes of an individual must sometimes be balanced against what is best for the community, so we will look at this in the OH context. In addition, there is a small but significant difference in the type of consent given to perform an intervention and that given for the release of personal information. I argue in this chapter that this means there are effectively *two* types of consenting processes at play in many of our OH activities, and discuss the relevance making this distinction more explicit in OH practice.

Chapter 4: Confidentiality.

In this chapter, I examine why confidentiality is so crucial in healthcare and OH practice. One of the reasons for its importance is that patients and workers entrust us with private and sensitive information. We should act in ways to merit that trust.

Another reason is that workers have a right to have their privacy respected. However, there are instances when the duty of confidentiality can (or even should) be breached, for example, if others might be harmed by non-disclosure. This confidentiality paradigm, with its allowed breaches, is arguably confusing for practitioners and patients/workers, and could *reduce* worker trust in OH. Nonetheless, this is the paradigm we usually work within, and I argue that if we are to be trusted by workers, then we must be open and transparent about the circumstances where confidentiality might be breached.

Chapter 5: Sickness absence

Although "sickness absence" is a very practical topic in OH, I have included this chapter in the "theory" section of this book. This is because I deal with the wider issues that can lead to sickness absence. For example, disadvantaged groups (such as the disabled) can be more likely to be absent from work through health problems. This leads to a discussion of the wider determinants of health, and how as a society we can treat vulnerable individuals more fairly. To advance this discussion, an awareness of the various theories of justice is helpful. A brief overview of such theories is presented. We then take a more in-depth look at my preferred option, the *capability approach*, which I believe is particularly appropriate in the OH context. I also argue that we have a special role, as OH professionals, in advising employers to have fair policies with regards to health, work and work attendance.

Chapter 6: Report writing

In this first of the "practical" chapters, a range of OH communications, mainly written, are described. The relevant ethical issues that they raise are highlighted. We thus see how in practice it can be difficult to balance all our ethical duties. For example, the duty to protect a worker's health *and* respecting his autonomy, or of respecting his confidentiality and right to privacy *and* giving the employer appropriate information. I describe four case vignettes, each being ethically problematic, to illustrate how these tensions and how they can be addressed. I explain my preferred courses of actions (with my justifications for these) in the examples described, but these are not definitive solutions. Indeed, there are rarely *absolutely correct* answers to many of our ethical dilemmas. However, I hope that by means of these examples, and the discussions that follow, you will feel more equipped to deal with similar ethical situations as they arise in your own OH practice.

Chapter 7: Health surveillance

Our primary aim as OH professionals is to protect the health of workers at work. Health surveillance is one activity *par excellence* that allows us to achieve this aim. If we use appropriate techniques to detect early health effects from workplace exposures, we can advise on appropriate actions to negate or minimize the harms to worker health, at individual and collective levels. However, for this approach to be effective, the health surveillance program must be designed on evidence-based criteria, conducted to good operational standards, and the results used effectively. Each of these steps bring some ethical challenges which are discussed in this chapter. Many of the ethical issues such as consent, confidentiality and autonomy are reviewed in this OH context.

Chapter 8: Vaccinations
In this third of the "practical" chapters, we look at ethical issues arising from vaccinations in the OH context. Most vaccinations are done as part of population health programs, so I will first compare and contrast the ethical issues arising in Public Health (PH) arena with those in OH. One question that challenges us in both areas of practice is whether it could ever be morally justifiable to coerce individuals into accepting to be vaccinated, especially in those situations when the main reason for vaccination might be to protect *others* in a community (PH) or patients (OH). I will argue that the answer to this may be dependent on how good the evidence for the protection of others through vaccination happens to be for that particular vaccine, by looking at the evidence-base for the influenza vaccination of health care workers.

Chapter 9: Conclusions
In this final chapter, we consider whether a framework for OH ethics might be possible, and if so, what it might look like. We look at the importance of learning from experience. I share one approach to ethical reflection which hopefully may be of help to some OH practitioners. We also consider what future changes in the world of work and OH may mean for OH ethics.

Part I
Theory

Chapter 2
The Doctor-Patient Relationship and Dual Obligations in Occupational Health

As OH professionals, we constantly interact with workers, managers and others. In this chapter, we will examine the ethical duties and obligations that we have towards these parties in our various OH roles. We will start by considering our relationship with our primary concern, the worker.

The Doctor-Patient Relationship

In the workplace, we may not always consider workers to be our "patients". However, for many of our OH roles and functions, our healthcare background can be crucial. In other roles and functions, it may be much less so, if at all. Nonetheless, it is likely that we are viewed as healthcare professionals, whatever the circumstances. It is important to bear this in mind, and to remember why workers and managers may be particularly respectful towards us, and at times entrust us with sensitive information. Our status as healthcare professionals carries with it some special responsibilities (usually specified by our regulatory bodies), and the professional relationships we form often presume (maybe subconsciously) the traditional "doctor-patient" relationship. Here, I use the phrase "doctor-patient" in a generic sense, to characterize *all* "healthcare professional-patient" relationships. I believe all such relationships share an important feature: The hallmark of these relationships is that they are based on **trust**.

In the context of the "traditional" (or therapeutic) doctor-patient relationship (DPR), it is said that patients need to trust doctors and other healthcare professionals, otherwise they would not come forward for their symptoms and conditions to be treated. Patient trust is also important for them to accept and follow the treatment and advice given to them by the healthcare professionals. Therefore, the importance of patient trust is justified by *consequentialist* arguments. Trust is necessary for patients to seek treatment, and for effective treatment to be delivered. The consequence of a lack of trust in healthcare professionals would be that the patients' conditions would be less effectively treated. The situation is not necessarily the same in OH practice

© Springer Nature Switzerland AG 2020
J. Tamin, *Occupational Health Ethics*,
https://doi.org/10.1007/978-3-030-47283-2_2

(I will separate out the different OH functions later in this chapter), but I believe that trust in OH professionals remains important. In Chap. 3 (when considering autonomy), I will put forward a further important reason for patients trusting healthcare (including OH) professionals.

Before we further consider trust in the OH context, let us first think about some important aspects of trust in the healthcare setting. Firstly, trust is rarely all or none. It may be greater or lesser according to which healthcare professional is involved with the patient, for what condition and in which circumstances. For example, it is suggested that a patient may generally trust his family practitioner more than a hospital doctor, but may trust the diagnosis of a cardiologist over that of his family practitioner, for his heart condition. Secondly, some argue that the *DPR* is now largely a myth, especially in the hospital setting. This is because the relationship is almost never just between one patient and one doctor, but more likely to be with a multitude of doctors, nurses, physiotherapists, and so on. Indeed, this situation mirrors OH practice, where multi-disciplinary teams work together to protect the health of workers. However, in both sets of circumstances, I do not believe that the importance of trust is eroded in any way. The emphasis should now be on each member, of a healthcare or OH team, being *individually* trustworthy, but there also needs to be *systemic* trustworthiness. The latter can only be achieved if organizations have policies, processes and procedures that ensure openness, transparency and good communication with workers or patients.

Let us now move from the general healthcare setting to considering workers' trust in OH professionals. Unfortunately, there is some evidence that a proportion of workers *mistrust* OH services, and by implication, OH professionals. What is different about OH in relation to trust? In order to answer this, over the remainder of this chapter we will explore the OH professional-worker relationship and our duties to various parties, which are occasionally in conflict, to see how these may affect worker trust, and what we may be able to do about this.

Dual Obligations

The reasons given by the workers who mistrust OH services include the fact that they felt the OH professional would be more on the side of the employer, or they were unsure how the OH professional would balance their obligations towards them (the workers) *vis a vis* their employers. Yet, the fact that we owe duties to workers *and* employers (and others) underpins the very **core** of what we are. So how do we reconcile these duties and gain (or retain) worker trust?

I believe that if we are to merit workers' trust in the face of conflicting obligations, we need to be open, honest and clear to all parties about what we do, and how we do it. But before we can be clear to others, we must first be clear *ourselves* about what we do (or ought to do), and how we do (or ought to do) this. And we need to be honest with ourselves about the tensions and difficulties we face, and understand why they arise, before we can find solutions to them.

We owe different obligations simultaneously to workers and employers. This has previously been described as "two-master ethics", and is now generally known as "dual obligations". Having dual obligations may not always be problematic, but when the interests of the two parties *do* come into conflict, then we can find ourselves in difficulty. Our best or most ethical approach in such situations could depend on the nature of the duties and obligations we owe to workers, employers and others, and which of these duties should take priority in those particular circumstances. Let us now consider these different duties in turn.

Duty to Workers

The primary purpose of OH is to protect the health of workers. Therefore, our primary duty to workers is to protect their health. This seems at first sight to be uncontroversial. However, this is not always the case, for example when we need to balance our duty to protect their health with our duty to respect their autonomy. We will look at this issue in greater depth in Chap. 3, when we discuss autonomy and consent. At this stage, I would like us to note the central importance of protecting the health of workers, as this gives us a bearing for our moral compass, when we encounter conflicts between our duties to workers and other parties. However, we must also be aware of conflicting duties even to the worker (such as protecting their health versus respecting their autonomy), that can arise on some occasions.

Given that most of us have a health background, the duty of protecting workers' health feels relatively straightforward and one to which we are happy to sign up to. We are used to having as the primary duty to our patients, caring for their lives and their health. Similarly, we respect the autonomy of patients in their healthcare choices, and avoid being paternalistic. In common with our duties in healthcare, we also owe workers a duty of confidentiality. This duty of confidentiality to patients is **not** absolute in therapeutic practice, as it can be breached if others might suffer harm from non-disclosure. Similarly, in OH practice we would keep worker information confidential, unless non-disclosure could result in harm to others. We will explore issues of disclosure and non-disclosure further in Chap. 4, when we look at privacy and confidentiality.

It seems reasonable to suggest that our duty to workers should largely mirror the healthcare professionals' duty to their patients. The use of the "four principles" in healthcare ethics, that is, respect for autonomy, nonmaleficence, beneficence and justice, and rules such as truth-telling and confidentiality, are likely to provide an equally appropriate framework in OH for our duty to workers. I believe this holds true for **most** of our OH practice, but there are times where OH is different to general healthcare in terms of ethical underpinning. I will elaborate on these differences later in this chapter, especially in the "OH Professional roles" section.

Duty to the Employer

We also owe duties to employers. Our main obligation towards them is to provide them with information and advice that allows them to discharge their health and safety responsibilities, that is to help them protect the health and safety of their workers. When viewed in this way, our primary duty to workers and to employers are in complete accord. However, in practice this may not be as straightforward. This is especially the case when an employer takes the stance of "I'm the one paying you. Give me the advice I want to hear!" Such an employer misses the point of OH. If we were to give biased and partial advice, we would go against our core values, and would lose the trust of the workforce. This would make it more difficult for us to protect the health of workers, and for employers to discharge their health and safety responsibilities in a meaningful way.

Whether we are paid directly by the employer or not should not matter. Neither should the fact that our contract with the employer may specify or not the requirement that our advice be honest, competent and impartial: this is at the core of what OH represents and should represent. The ICOH ethics guidance *does* recommend that we have a clause on ethics in our contracts, and I would strongly endorse this. But even if this clause is not in our current contracts, this does not absolve us from doing what is professionally and ethically the correct thing to do, which is to be honest and impartial in giving our advice to the employer. For example, some authors point out that the fact that we owe obligations to employers does **not** mean that we can provide them with information merely based on this, without a consideration of the worker's right to confidentiality and consent (permission to disclose). I agree with them and I will elaborate further on permission to disclose and confidentiality in Chaps. 3 and 4 respectively. It is important for employers and workers to understand that this is our ethical stance. Although some employers may not like this, it is essential for us to practice in this manner if we want workers to trust OH professionals and OH services.

As OH professionals, we also owe a duty of confidence *to* the employer. In particular, we must keep commercially sensitive information confidential, except if keeping this information confidential could result in harm to others, whether to workers or to members of the community. We should first raise our concerns with the relevant senior managers and comply with internal procedures for raising these concerns (keeping records of having done so). However, if our concerns are not heeded, and the risk of harm to workers or members of the community remains significant, then we need to alert the competent authorities (known as "whistleblowing"). If we are faced with this difficult situation, it would be wise to discuss with a senior colleague and with our medical defense insurer (or equivalent), for advice. For their part, the employer may insist that we owe them a duty of confidence. They should be reminded that this duty is not absolute. We need to balance this duty against our first and foremost ethical (and in most jurisdictions, legal as well) duty, which is to **protect the health and safety** of workers, and if members of the community might be at risk, then we also have a duty to protect their health and safety. This is the moral justification for breaching our duty of confidentiality to the employer. Hopefully, this would be a rare occurrence.

Duty to Other Parties

Although we owe obligations **primarily** to workers and employers, we also owe obligations to other stakeholders, such as pension fund trustees, or "the public" (such as when public safety may be at risk), at various times. So, in practice our obligations are often "multiple" rather than just "dual". However, I will continue to use the term "dual obligation", as it is the one in common use, but recognizing that we often owe obligations to more than the two main stakeholders.

When we consider the obligations owed to third parties that may be harmed in some way (for example, by a patient), then such a situation also exists in the healthcare setting. For example, in a therapeutic setting, a nurse could be made aware of a safeguarding issue, and he will then have a duty to keep the vulnerable party safe; or a neurologist might become aware that her patient with uncontrolled epilepsy continues to drive, in which case she would have a duty to other road users placed at risk of death or injury from her patient. This duty to those who might be harmed seems no different then, whether in healthcare or OH practice. I think this is correct. However, what differentiates professionals in healthcare settings from those with dual obligations, is likely to be the *frequency* with which this concern for third parties arises out of their practice. In addition, there may be a difference of *emphasis*. What I mean by this, is the fact that healthcare professionals rightly make their patient their **first** concern. It then follows that any other consideration (including public safety), necessarily then becomes secondary to this. I accept that this needs some qualification, as the risk of third party death or serious injury does require the healthcare professional to re-balance the priorities in their obligations.

Another way of looking at the balance of these priorities would be to consider the situation of the public health (PH) doctor. She would have the health of society or a community, as her primary concern. She would still have regard to whether any PH initiative or policy might harm or disadvantage some individuals, for example, but this would not be her primary focus. This could then be viewed as being at the opposite end of the spectrum compared with the "treating doctor" (as illustrated in Fig. 2.1). Figure 2.1 illustrates the continuum between the two sets of obligations (y-axis) and the two "extremes" of the doctor role (x-axis). OH professionals would then find themselves somewhere in between the "treating doctor" and the "PH doctor" positions on the x-axis. I believe this is a reasonable portrayal of the fact that as OH professionals, we tend to remain more aware (compared with healthcare professionals in a therapeutic setting) of our obligations to other parties, even when we are interacting with the individual worker. This difference in approach can sometimes be seen when there are divergences of opinion between the treating doctor and OH professionals. These divergent opinions can arise when it comes to assessing the risk

Fig. 2.1 Continuum of obligations owed to the individual patient versus society by different doctors (and other healthcare professionals)

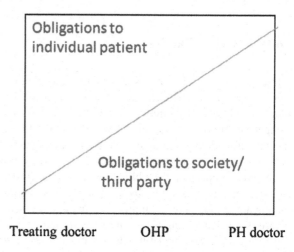

of allowing a patient/worker with some residual risk of an incapacitating condition, returning to *safety critical* work. For example, a cardiologist may feel that her patient, on treatment for a heart condition, can return to work as a train driver, given the low risk of a sudden incapacitating event. The OH professional, on the other hand, may be more cautious in that regard, and recommend a more stringent risk assessment given the serious consequences to public safety if such an incapacity *did* occur. Thus, although in theory **both** the cardiologist and the OH professional have obligations towards the patient **and** the public, in practice there is often a difference in how these obligations are discharged. I suggest that generally, OH professionals are more sensitive to their duties to the public, especially where public safety might be at risk.

Another aspect in which OH professionals differ from other healthcare professionals is that we retain obligations to other parties (such as employers, pension funds) even when there is **no** risk of harm to third parties. These arise from an intrinsic aspect of our role, which is to provide unbiased advice on a worker's health in relation to work. Such advice includes fitness for work reports to employers and ill-health retirement reports to pension funds. This aspect of third party obligation, which does *not* require the need for harm to others for its existence, differentiates OH (and possibly other "dual obligation" specialties) from mainstream healthcare. Therefore, although our primary focus is protecting the health of workers, we may have more (compared with other healthcare professionals) explicit obligations to other parties, which in turn may lead to more ethical tensions when these obligations are in conflict.

A Fiduciary Relationship?

In addition to *trust* being central to the DPR (and by analogy, to the healthcare professional-patient relationship), an important feature of that relationship is said to be the *power imbalance* between the two parties. This asymmetrical relationship arises, for example, from the vulnerability of the patient, and the knowledge and expertise of the doctor (or other healthcare professional). Trust and a power imbalance are the necessary requirements for a *fiduciary* relationship between the two parties.

There is strong support for the DPR to be viewed as a fiduciary one. I agree with that view, and by extension, I would consider healthcare professional-patient relationships in therapeutic settings to be fiduciaries and patients to be the "vulnerable parties". Given the power imbalance between the two parties, there is general agreement that such a relationship would then impose certain obligations on the fiduciary (that is, the healthcare professional). These are: no conflicts of interest, the fiduciary should not profit from that relationship, and the fiduciary owes a duty of confidentiality and a duty of undivided loyalty to the patient. One should note that even in a therapeutic relationship, there is a *caveat* to the duty of undivided loyalty, that is, it would be breached if there were the risk of third party harm. Apart from that exception, the obligations to patients seem reasonable, and resonate well with our experience as healthcare professionals. This also applies to much of our OH work. There are however, some of our OH roles where a fiduciary relationship would be problematic, and we will consider this in the next section.

Independence

Some OH roles or functions require us to be *independent*. However, independence can be interpreted in various ways. For example, ICOH's Code of Ethics repeatedly emphasizes the importance of OH professionals having "full professional independence". In this context, this full professional independence is required in order to protect the health and safety of workers (our primary purpose), and OH professionals should not be influenced by any party in making that type of judgement and giving that type of advice. This seems to me to be uncontroversial. At least, that is how it *ought* to be. It is possible that one party or another might try to put pressure on the OH professional for her to change her opinion or advice. This is where maintaining one's professional integrity is crucial, and why ICOH's stance on professional independence is so important.

Similarly, there are national codes that stress the importance of professional independence in healthcare settings, and again, the justification is that the health of the patient should come first. Such requirements for professional independence, to protect patient or worker **health**, are entirely compatible with a *fiduciary* healthcare professional-patient relationship.

However, what about the circumstances where the healthcare professional needs to be independent *from* the patient or worker? In the UK, this situation arises when an OH physician assesses eligibility for early retirement on health grounds, for some major public pension schemes, where there is a statutory (that is, legal) requirement for *independence*. Here, the OH professional is required to be independent from the employer *and* the worker (or applicant). Therefore, in this capacity, the OH professional would not be able to fulfill all fiduciary obligations, especially the "duty of undivided loyalty", and remain independent from the worker/applicant at the same time. So, how can we reconcile these diametrically opposed obligations of the OH professional in this scenario?

OH Professional Roles

One approach to resolving these incompatible demands on the OH professional would be to separate out the roles that she undertakes, and to clearly specify which role she is fulfilling at any given time. The two roles that I would specify here are the "quasi-therapeutic" and the "independent" roles. I accept that it is possible to describe other OH roles, but as the two I am describing are at the extreme opposite ends of the spectrum of OH roles, this gives us a good starting point.

Given that our main priority is to protect the health of workers, I believe the "quasi-therapeutic" role sits well with OH professionals. I use the term *quasi*-therapeutic because in many countries, OH professionals do **not** provide the full range of therapeutic services (on the other hand, in other countries primary care and OH services are combined). However, even in the countries where full treatment services are not provided, OH professionals are often arguably still involved in some forms of treatment such as emergency first aid, immunizations, advice and counselling, and referrals to physiotherapy or psychological services. With such interactions between workers and OH professionals, there may be little, if any, difference compared with interactions in a therapeutic setting, especially in terms of mutual trust.

In contrast, in the scenario where independence from the worker is required, as in the case of assessing a worker/applicant for ill-health retirement (IHR), then the OH professional in such a role would be best described as "independent". There is still the need for some degree of trust, for example, it is better if the worker can trust the OH professional to be unbiased and fair. Furthermore, it is important that the OH professional be competent at performing this assessment, and know the detailed requirements of the pension scheme, as well as the functional requirements of the job that the applicant states he can no longer do. However, it is probably difficult for most applicants to know whether the OH professional is indeed competent and fair. So, while the OH professional is performing the assessment, it would be helpful if she could be open and transparent about the issues under consideration, be they features of the relevant medical condition(s), the job or alternative jobs, and the pension scheme rules. This would probably help to demonstrate fairness, competence and thoroughness to the applicant. Nonetheless, it is still possible that an applicant who is unsuccessful at securing the financial benefits he was hoping for, to feel aggrieved, and even question the OH professional's competence and/or impartiality. In those circumstances, although we might have preferred that the encounter (that is, the assessment) be conducted with some degree of mutual trust, we have to accept that this will not always be possible, but the assessment can still proceed regardless. I must stress that in **all** OH roles, whether quasi-therapeutic or independent, we must retain full *professional* independence, (as is stated in the ICOH code of ethics).

The relative importance of trust in the relationships and interactions we have just been considering are summarized in the above table. The central importance of trust is highlighted in the therapeutic setting, between healthcare professional and patient. Similarly, in the OH quasi-therapeutic role, it is important that workers trust us, so that we can fulfill our primary role, which is to protect their health. It is more likely that they will accept our advice on health risks from work exposures, advice on prevention, and such like, if this trust exists. However, the *level* of trust may not need to be quite as high as in the truly therapeutic setting (where the level of trust is usually very high indeed). In our independent OH role, it would still be desirable to have the worker (or applicant to pension fund, in the example I have described) trusting us as being competent and impartial. I have suggested that by being open and transparent about our decision making and advice, we are more likely to engender some trust. However, it is still possible to carry out the required assessment even if this trust is lacking.

In therapeutic settings, a significant power imbalance between healthcare professional and patient is usually in evidence. The vulnerability of the patient, at a time of distress from his symptoms, or worries about the cause of his symptoms, or lack of familiarity with the therapeutic setting (such as a hospital) puts him at a significant disadvantage. The healthcare professional, on the other hand, will have familiarity with the context of that therapeutic encounter, greater knowledge about the condition and its implications, and usually greater authority because of her status. It is true that there are occasions where this power imbalance can be overstated, for example, when the patient has greater knowledge of his condition (or thinks he has, after doing internet searches). Nonetheless, in the majority of healthcare professional-patient encounters, the healthcare professional is in the dominant role. It is likely that OH quasi-therapeutic encounters largely mirror this power imbalance, mainly because of the OH professional's knowledge, expertise and status. However, a worker may not always be in a distressed and vulnerable state, for example, if the OH encounter is for a routine procedure, such as health surveillance (assuming the worker is already very familiar with the procedure). If a worker were attending an OH consultation because of suffering physical or psychological symptoms, then he would probably be just as vulnerable as in a truly therapeutic encounter. In an independent OH assessment, a power imbalance can arise because the worker (or applicant) is dependent on the OH professional's opinion or decision as to whether, for example, the pension scheme criteria for ill-health retirement are met. It is also likely that the OH professional's status and expertise will also confer further "power". However, there are also occasions (hopefully rare) where the OH professional can feel threatened and intimidated by the applicant or their representative. In these circumstances, one could argue that the power imbalance is, in fact, reversed.

Lastly in Table 2.1, we compare the fiduciary obligations that may or may not arise in the three types of interactions. As previously mentioned, the healthcare professional-patient relationship in a therapeutic setting shares all the hallmarks of a fiduciary relationship. This relationship places on the fiduciary (the healthcare professional), the obligations of having no conflicts of interest, not profiting from her position, a duty of confidence and a duty of undivided loyalty. I have suggested that in the quasi-therapeutic OH role, OH professionals should have similar obligations derived from the fiduciary relationship. The duty of undivided loyalty may sit slightly uncomfortably with us, given that we also owe duties to the employer and other parties. However, if we remember that in our quasi-therapeutic role, our *primary* purpose is the health of workers. This is not dissimilar from the therapeutic situation, where the healthcare professional would have as her *primary* focus, the health of her patients. There are still obligations owed to others, especially when they might be at risk of harm. So, although the "undivided" needs to be qualified in this way, I think we can feel comfortable that in most situations, be it in a healthcare or OH quasi-therapeutic role, our loyalty should be towards the patient or worker.

However, in the OH independent role, we need to be independent *from* the worker, so we cannot owe any loyalty to the worker/applicant, let alone *undivided* loyalty. As we cannot be independent from *and* loyal to a party, these two duties are incompatible if we try to action them *simultaneously*. It makes more sense to say that in the independent role, an OH professional cannot be in a fiduciary relationship with the worker/applicant. This does not absolve the independent OH role from the other obligations (namely having no conflicts of interest, not profiting from their position and owing a duty of confidence). But the OH professional does **not** owe a worker undivided loyalty in the independent role. I think it is important to have this clear in our own minds, and then we can be open and transparent about this situation when we communicate to workers, or other applicants we may be assessing, in this independent role as in others.

I will return to the above distinction between our roles later, by looking at how this affects the report-writing process in practice (in Chap. 6, "Report writing"). At this point, I want to emphasize the importance of being clear and transparent to workers about how our role (either quasi-therapeutic or independent) affects our relationship with them, as I believe this can help towards improving workers' trust in OH professionals.

Concurrent Primary Care and OH Functions

The question I would like to consider here is: could the same healthcare professional provide primary care *and* an OH functions at the same time? This is the current practice in some countries. In other countries, this approach is discouraged on the

Table 2.1 Comparison of Trust, Power imbalance and Fiduciary obligations in the therapeutic healthcare professional-patient, "quasi-therapeutic" OH professional-worker and independent OH professional-worker relationships

	Therapeutic healthcare professional-patient relationship	Quasi-therapeutic OH Professional-worker	Independent OH Professional-worker
Trust	+++	+	±
Power imbalance	++	+	±
Fiduciary obligations	++	+	**Incompatible** with "duty of undivided loyalty"

basis that the two functions have inherent ethical conflicts of interest. In some dual obligation settings, such as military medicine, this happens by necessity.

Those who regard the two functions, if practiced concurrently, as being necessarily in conflict point out that an OH professional providing primary care will need full and extensive patient information to provide effective treatment. If she is later to communicate with her patient's employer in an OH capacity, she cannot "un-know" that patient information. The patient/worker trust she gained in the former (primary care) function could in effect be breached in performing the latter (OH) one. This seems to be the nub of the problem.

However, if trust is based on honesty, transparency and clarity of our roles (as I have previously argued), then I believe this apparent ethical conflict can be resolved. We have at the outset to communicate clearly with our patient/worker about our *dual* role. The OH role that we should later be able to perform is the *quasi-therapeutic* one, and **not** the *independent* one. The trust demands of a therapeutic primary care relationship and a quasi-therapeutic OH relationship are not dissimilar, as the OH professional has fiduciary obligations to the patient/worker similar to those of a primary care doctor to her patient. This is very different to the "independent OH professional-worker" situations, which **cannot** be based on a fiduciary relationship (see Table 2.1). For example, the differences in the OH roles and functions manifest themselves when we give advice to the employer to protect the patient/worker's health (quasi-therapeutic role), as opposed to advice on the patient/worker's eligibility to IHR benefits (independent role). I therefore see a concurrent primary care and quasi-therapeutic OH role as being compatible, but **not** a concurrent primary care role with an independent OH role.

Conclusion

In OH, our "dual obligations" to workers, employers and others should play a major, if not pivotal, role in our ethics paradigm. We need to balance our duties to all these parties all the time. This may sound like walking a tightrope constantly, but in practice this need not always be the case. Although we should always be aware of these obligations to different parties, the obligations do not necessarily come into conflict on each occasion. Indeed, it could be argued that one of the skills OH professionals should develop is *reducing* the conflict when this occurs. We are more likely to achieve this if we are trusted by all parties.

Nonetheless, our primary purpose is to protect the health of workers. Therefore, *workers'* trust in OH professionals is of central importance to us. Unfortunately, there is evidence that workers do *not* always trust OH professionals. I suggest that this could be improved by being transparent and open about how we balance our duties to different parties. The approach I have suggested is to be clear and explicit about which OH role we are undertaking at any given time. When we are performing a *quasi-therapeutic* role, our primary duty is to the worker. However, in an *independent* role, our primary duty is to the commissioner of that assessment (such as an employer or a pension fund manager). It would also be helpful if our regulators, for example through their codes of practice, explicitly recognized the difference in these roles. This would reduce workers' **confusion** (which was an important contributor, in the studies I previously mentioned, to workers mistrusting OH) about how we balance our obligations, and this I believe would improve worker trust in our services. If workers trusted OH services more, this would in turn enhance our ability to protect their health. (For an illustration of this latter point, see the 'Relational autonomy' section in Chap. 3).

Chapter 3
Consent

Introduction

Consent is a fundamental concept in healthcare ethics. As healthcare professionals, the mere thought that we might treat patients without their consent is unacceptable, and to treat them against their wishes would be abhorrent to us. Indeed, in many jurisdictions, such non-consensual actions would constitute an assault and a battery on the patient. Yet, I believe that it is not so much the threat of legal censure that most of us worry about. In my view, it is our deep respect for patient dignity that stops us from acting without the patient's full agreement. We chose to work in health care because we share such values, which were then further developed in us by our professional training. So, it is not surprising that we carry the same respect for the patient's wishes into our OH practice. But what is the moral justification for the concept of consent?

Origins of Consent

In biomedical ethics, the importance of consent was first formally articulated following the Nuremberg trials, following the horrors of Nazi experimentation on their prisoners. The Nuremberg Code was developed to ensure that it would no longer be possible to conduct research on human beings without their full understanding and agreement. The primary concerns at that time were to prevent the coercion of, and harm to, human research subjects (now more properly termed "participants"). That is, it was thought to be important to ensure *voluntariness* of research participants and protecting their *bodily integrity*. In due course, the concept of consent was extended to also cover therapeutic encounters. In addition, it came to reflect the respect we have for a patient's (or research participant's) **autonomy**.

© Springer Nature Switzerland AG 2020
J. Tamin, *Occupational Health Ethics*,
https://doi.org/10.1007/978-3-030-47283-2_3

Autonomy

Our ability to determine how we live our lives, that is, to be autonomous beings, is of critical importance to us. Autonomy has also become of central importance in moral philosophy. However, it has been pointed out that there is more than one definition or understanding of autonomy, so some commentators have suggested that autonomy might not deserve its pre-eminence in contemporary moral philosophy. Nonetheless, in the fields of healthcare and OH practice autonomy has become and remains a pivotal concept, as it is closely aligned to *patient* autonomy (as opposed to the previously prevailing *paternalistic* medical ethics).

It would still be useful to reflect further on what we mean when we say that we should *respect autonomy* in OH practice. If acting autonomously means that we are acting in a way that reflects our values and beliefs, then we need to give some thought as to which choice or action is *actually* in line with these values, that is, which choice would make us *truly* "self-determining". It is not necessarily the first thought or choice that comes to us. Rather, we need to consider which choice, decision or action would be more aligned to our core values. This form of autonomy has been described as *reflective* autonomy. Although it may be thought of as a rather idealistic view of autonomy, I believe that it is the version that we should at least aspire to. I would go further than this. If we make a choice that is *not* aligned to our deepest values and beliefs, then that choice does reflect who we are as a person, and we are **not** really acting autonomously.

Trust and Autonomy

In the previous chapter, we saw how important trust is in the health care context. It is also crucially important that workers trust us (as OH professionals), although they may not necessarily always be entrusting us with their lives and health (as they would in a therapeutic context). We also recognize the importance of patient (or worker) autonomy. However, trust and autonomy are concepts that do not necessarily sit comfortably together. Autonomy focusses on the *individual's* right to choose and to self-determine. Trust necessarily involves *more* than one individual. Of course, it is possible for a patient to make an autonomous decision and to trust the advice of a healthcare professional at the same time. But it could be argued that increasing patient autonomy may be at the expense of the trust between patient and healthcare professional: if the patient can make his own decision, then it matters little whether he trusts the doctor or nurse, or not.

Relational Autonomy

However, although autonomy and trust might in some ways diverge at conceptual level, this may not necessarily be problematic in practice.

Consider for example, Albert, a worker whose health is deteriorating as a result of some harmful workplace exposure. His OH adviser, Allison, recommends to him that he should avoid further exposure. She suggests writing to his manager to advise that he be redeployed away from that area of exposure. However, he is concerned that he may lose his job instead. He has seen this happen previously with colleagues in similar situations. He does not give consent for this advice to go to his manger. He has carefully considered the effects of losing his income, his ability to feed and care for his family, so he is prepared to risk his health. On the face of it, this is an autonomous choice. Without consent, Allison cannot disclose information to his manager (let us assume that no other factors come into play, such as a risk to other workers, which we will consider later in Chap. 7). Whether he trusts Allison a lot, or a little, or not at all, seems at first sight to be of little import to his decision.

But let us imagine that he *does* trust Allison. Within this relationship of trust, she is more able to reflect more deeply *with* him the full consequences of his initial choice. Albert is a proud man, and wants to remain self-sufficient and be able to raise his family in the best way he can. Should his health deteriorate much further, this will become impossible for him to achieve, as he would end up having to give up his job due to chronic ill-health. We can imagine that, as a result of this further reflection, he is more likely to decide to follow Allison's advice in order to protect his health.

This not uncommon scenario in OH practice demonstrates how a relationship of trust can *enhance* autonomous choices. This worker finally made the choice more closely aligned with his own values. It also illustrates the fact that "no man is an island". We exercise our autonomy within social contexts, including healthcare and the work environment. This more enlightened conception of autonomy is described as *relational* autonomy. Thus, trust matters in healthcare and OH practice, not only for the reasons discussed in Chap. 2, but also because it can promote greater patient and worker autonomy. This is a further important reason why I believe healthcare and OH practitioners should do their utmost to be trustworthy.

Solidarity

I mentioned in the previous paragraph that most of us live and work within communities and societies. It can be argued that it is the community and societal arrangements that give us the opportunity to exercise our autonomy. In turn, we can recognize this and reciprocate by choosing to act in *solidarity* with our community, be it our family, fellow workers or wider society. That is, we choose to act in ways that express our shared commitment to the common good.

Therefore, in Albert's case, had there were the possibility that his initial decision not to allow Allison to inform the manager of the harmful health effects of the exposure could have affected fellow workers (in this example I had suggested it would not), then he might have changed his mind out of solidarity for them. Of course, there is the additional issue of whether the possibility of harm to others should trump his consent in any case, but we will consider that line of argument later under "Informed consent".

Solidarity is an ethical concept used in Public Health ethics, but so far it has not been often (and in my view, sufficiently) used in OH ethical analysis. After all, in OH we look after groups of workers as well as the individual worker. Therefore, it is useful to think about solidarity in certain ethical situations (for example, see Chap. 8), and to remember that although autonomy is a very important consideration, it is not the only one. On the other hand, it does not mean that autonomy and solidarity need to be in conflict. When we understand autonomy in relational terms, that is, thinking how our choices and decisions could affect others in our community, this describes a richer version of autonomy. This relational approach recognizes the importance of both, autonomy and solidarity. Indeed, in this paradigm, they become mutually co-dependent and reinforcing.

What Does This Mean for Consent?

We saw earlier that consent is required because we want to respect Albert's autonomy. What we understand *autonomy* to be is therefore important to our understanding of consent. I have argued that a narrow, individualistic conception of autonomy does not bear close scrutiny. We would hope that Albert would at least reflect on his decision in terms what self-determination means for him, and think of the consequences for his family, colleagues and the wider community. Allison can help him with his deliberations, assuming there is a relationship of trust between them. However, despite these further reflections, it is still possible that Albert might not consent for Allison to disclose relevant information and advice to his manager. As I mentioned above, I believe that Allison should **not** act without his consent, except if there were a risk of harm to others (see later). There is some irony in this: The reason for needing Albert's consent for Allison to write to his manager is to *protect him from harm.* Yet if he refuses to give consent, that choice *will* probably lead to deterioration of his health, as he will continue to be exposed to the harmful exposure (and remember the primary aim of OH is to protect the health of workers!). Allison will realize this and will probably experience inner turmoil from the ethical conflict between the need to respect Albert's autonomy on the one hand, *and* protecting him from harm (principle of beneficence, as well as being the OH primary purpose) on the other. However, choosing beneficence over autonomy would be considered being paternalistic, which is generally not viewed as acceptable. One *caveat* to this are the instances where the health deterioration could be life threatening. The question then could arise as to what degree (and severity) of risk is needed to override consent. These instances when consent for disclosure is refused often lead to difficult ethical tensions, and Allison should also discuss Albert's case (preferably anonymizing his details) with an experienced colleague.

However, the benefit of understanding the concepts of *reflective* autonomy is that Albert has a better chance of making a choice aligned with his deeply held values (which hopefully will include his recognition of his *solidarity* with others, including his co-workers); and of *relational* autonomy (in a relationship of trust) is that it allows Allison to help him with that reflection. Although this further reflection does not necessarily guarantee the best *health* outcome for Albert (if he still refuses to consent), at least this understanding gives Allison the chance to act in the best way she can in these circumstances.

Informed Consent

So far, I have used the term "consent". However, the commonly used phrase is "informed consent". Some point out that "informed consent" is a tautology, as consent is not real if it is not *informed*. To some extent, I do agree with them. But in general, I prefer to use the phrase "informed consent" rather than simply "consent" for three reasons. Firstly, it is the phrase generally used in the ethico-legal literature. Secondly, it reminds how important the role of *information* is in the context of obtaining consent. Thirdly, when we use the term "consent", I believe that we could be describing either of **two** consent processes, or both; the two consent processes being *informed consent* and *permission to disclose*.

I will explain what I mean by these two processes, using health surveillance as an example. The ICOH code does highlight the importance of obtaining informed consent for health surveillance. It emphasizes, for example, the need to explain the possible positive and negative consequences of participating in this activity, as part of the consenting process. I agree with this, but also feel that this needs further elaboration.

Consider the case of Billy, a battery worker working in an environment where he is exposed to lead dust and fumes. His health surveillance will include biomonitoring, which typically consists of taking a blood sample to measure his serum lead levels (and sometimes a full blood count and zinc protoporphyrin as well). He attends the OH clinic for this blood test. Now, a word of caution. It might be thought that the fact that he attends voluntarily for this blood test, or even offers his arm for the venepuncture, is evidence of *implied* or *tacit* consent. I would discourage reliance on this. As mentioned previously, consent without information is **not** real or valid consent. Kathryn, the OH adviser needs to explain at least the *purpose* of taking the blood sample, that is, to test for blood lead, as high blood levels of lead would harm his health. She needs to reassure him that it will not be tested for anything else without his knowledge and agreement (such as blood alcohol). He needs to know *who* will be given the result, and what the consequences might be. For example, if the level is high, he may be moved temporarily to another area. Sometimes this may have a negative financial impact if he were not able to work as much overtime. Such arrangements are often agreed between management and trade union representatives, but it should not be assumed that Billy knows what they are. If his blood lead level is very high, he may need to be suspended from all work involving lead exposure until his lead levels are satisfactory. Of course, the health surveillance process is for Billy's protection, but he needs to understand that there can be negative consequences as well. In addition, should he have any other questions about this blood test that I have not mentioned here, Kathryn must answer these truthfully and to the best of her knowledge.

The information that must be provided to Billy is therefore wide-ranging, sometimes specific, sometimes in-depth, according to his needs. It must also be provided in a language that is clear and understandable to him. Only then can this part of the consenting process be truly *informed* consent.

Then there is a second part to the consenting process, which occurs when the blood test result is available. This will then be disclosed, with Billy's consent (I use the term generically here) to the relevant parties, such as his manager or a Health and Safety manager. I separate this second consent (for disclosure of the result) from the *informed consent* part of the consent process, and term this as a *permission to disclose* process. I will explain the differences between informed consent and permission to disclose, in the next section.

Permission to Disclose

When Billy's blood test result is available, Kathryn will send this information to appropriate parties, such as his manager, and the occupational hygienist, for example. This disclosure of Billy's information also needs his consent. This is what I would term *permission to disclose*, and this is **separate** from informed consent.

To obtain his permission to disclose, Kathryn still needs to inform Billy what the result is, *to whom* she proposes to send it to, and *what* information will be disclosed (for example, sometimes blood lead results are disclosed in bands A, B, C etc. rather than the actual numerical result). She would also need to explain the possible consequences if he declined permission for this to be disclosed. Still, the information that Billy needs at the stage of obtaining *permission to disclose* is much more limited in scope, compared with the level of information that Kathryn required to give him to obtain his *informed consent*, as I described previously. Moreover, this part of the consenting process protects Billy's *privacy* (the result is his private information), as well as his autonomy. He still makes an autonomous choice, as he can agree or not to give his permission. Indeed, I previously used the example of Albert choosing whether to allow his health information to be disclosed (which was therefore another permission to disclose scenario), to illustrate the importance of Allison respecting his choices, therefore respecting his autonomy. Informed consent primarily protects autonomy, whereas permission to disclose protects privacy **and** autonomy.

Conflation of the Term "Consent"

In non-OH healthcare settings, patients give informed consent to undergo therapeutic interventions. Permission to disclose is rarely required in comparison, but would occur when a medical report is written, or patient data is used for purposes other than patient care. However, the instances when either form of consent is required tend to be discrete and separate events. On the other hand, in OH practice, there tends to be some form of report or information disclosure to a non-clinical party following most interventions (such as for biomonitoring) or assessments (such as a fitness to work evaluation). Thus, the need for the need for both informed consent and permission to disclose *simultaneously*, occurs more often in OH practice than in other healthcare settings. This is probably the reason why a small, but significant, difference between the two types of consent has the potential for creating more confusion in OH practice than elsewhere.

Let us look again at the consenting requirements in Billy's case. For Kathryn to take the blood sample, Billy's informed consent is essential. Without this, Kathryn cannot proceed, otherwise it would constitute an act of assault and battery in many jurisdictions. It would be equally reprehensible from a moral perspective. Once his blood lead result is known, Kathryn needs to obtain Billy's permission to disclose this result. If she were to do this without his permission, the breach of his privacy would **not** constitute an assault or battery. This does *not* mean that she should ignore his decision whether to permit disclosure or not. Harm can still result from breaches of privacy, such as psychological injury or economic loss. However, the types of harm are likely to be different to situations where informed consent is required, where physical harm is also a possibility.

It is true that Kathryn could obtain "consent" at the same time for both, taking the blood sample *and* disclosing the result later. I would suggest that this is not good practice. It conflates the two types of consent, which can lead to confusion, at least at conceptual level. For example, if Kathryn did disclose the blood result against his wish, she might mistakenly be thought of having actioned an assault (because of acting without "consent"). Also, if she did not know the result *before* taking the blood test (which she would clearly not), then it could be argued that this crucial information would be missing when she were obtaining Billy's informed consent. But, without this information, could his consent really be *informed*? The confusions arise because we conflate the concepts "informed consent" and "permission to disclose" if we use the term "consent" or "informed consent" to mean *both* interchangeably. If we use different terminology to explain the reason for consent, that is, either for an intervention (informed consent) *or* for a disclosure (permission to disclose), then such confusion is avoided.

However, one could argue that Billy's example is not very realistic. Why would he refuse permission to disclose the blood test result, having initially consented to having his blood taken? I agree that this would seem unlikely (although it may happen on occasions). I used this example to illustrate the two separate types of consent required for much OH work, such as health surveillance and fitness for work assessments, with subsequent information that needs to be communicated to managers.

Let us then consider a more realistic scenario where conflation of the concepts is relevant. Charles, a nurse, sustains a needlestick injury. The donor patient, Elaine, is thought to be at high risk of being HIV positive. Charles is considering taking post-exposure prophylaxis (PEP) but is aware that there are possible serious side-effects from this medication. He would therefore prefer to know whether Elaine is in fact HIV positive, rather than take PEP that he might not need. On the other hand, if Elaine is HIV positive, then he would take PEP as he feels the benefits from this would clearly outweigh the risks.

In the first scenario, Elaine's HIV status is not known, and she would need a blood test to determine this. Her *informed consent* is required to proceed to taking this sample. If she refuses, no blood sample can be taken, as otherwise proceeding without consent would constitute an assault.

The second scenario is that Elaine has previously been tested, and her HIV status is in her hospital file. In order for Charles to obtain this information, her *permission to disclose* is required. If she refuses to give Charles (or the OH department, on Charles' behalf) this permission, the situation is still difficult. This is because to proceed without her permission would be breaching her right to **privacy**. This is still a very important interest to be protected. However, in balancing this against the harm that Charles would suffer if the information is not disclosed (whether she is HIV positive or negative), the case could be made that disclosure without permission is justifiable. At the very least, this situation allows us to *balance* the moral arguments from both sides. This is very different to the first scenario, where to proceed without informed consent would mean committing an assault, and there is therefore **no** possibility of weighing up the moral arguments in that first scenario.

This example thus illustrates a practical consequence of making a clear distinction between informed consent and permission to disclose.

Capacity

Although I have been pointing out the *differences* between informed consent and permission to disclose so far, they also share much in common. In both situations, there should no *coercion* on the worker to give consent or permission. Another important feature common to both is that the worker should be able to *understand* the information given to them by the OH professional. This presumes that the worker has the *capacity* to understand this information, and is *competent* to make their autonomous decision, for example, whether to consent or not.

Those who are usually deemed to have insufficient capacity for such decisions include children and those who suffer from very severe mental impairment. Therefore, the instances in OH practice where we need to consider capacity in the workplace may be thought to be rare. However, OH colleagues have pointed out to me that individuals with very severe learning disabilities are increasingly in employment, which is very welcome. As with any other worker, we need to make sure that he or she understands what a procedure entails in order to give their informed consent, say, for venepuncture or vaccination, or permission to disclose a report or result.

In this section, I will briefly list some of the general principles which should apply when we are thinking of capacity and competence. Firstly, we should presume that someone *does* have capacity unless we have good evidence of the contrary. Secondly, individuals can have capacity in *some* areas of their lives, and not others. Thirdly, if we deem that they do not have capacity in the area where we need their consent, then *we* should **not** be making that decision for them. There should be someone in the role of *guardian*, who would make that decision on their behalf, and that decision should be in their *best interest*.

I will later mention again this issue of capacity, in practical OH situations, namely in the contexts of report writing (Chap. 6) and of health surveillance (Chap. 7).

Conclusion

It is essential to obtain the *informed consent* of workers before any intervention, such as venepuncture, immunizations or assessments. This shows that we respect their autonomy. At its best, autonomy is reflective and represents the choice most aligned to the worker's deeply held values. That choice will also hopefully take account of his relationship with others, including his colleagues and his community.

In OH practice, we also communicate results (that is, personal data) and reports (on individual workers) to the employer. These communications must also be done with the worker's consent. I have described this form of consent as *permission to disclose*, which recognizes and protects *privacy*, as well as autonomy.

Chapter 4
Confidentiality

Whatever, in connection with my professional practice or not, in connection with it, I see or hear, in the life of men, which ought not to be spoken of abroad, I will not divulge, as reckoning that all such should be kept secret. (Hippocrates).

Confidentiality and Healthcare

Confidentiality is one of the most important ethical requirements in healthcare. It has been described as "one of the most venerable moral obligations of medical ethics", and "central to the therapeutic relationship". Confidentiality is also said to be "enshrined in all codes of medical ethics".

Why is confidentiality so important in healthcare? The primary justification for patient confidentiality is that without assurances that their sensitive information would not be unnecessarily disclosed, patients might not seek healthcare professional help and advice. Or they might not disclose all their symptoms, or relevant information to the healthcare professional, which might lead to sub-optimal care and treatment. This is therefore a consequence-based justification. Other justifications for maintaining patient confidentiality are duty-based (confidentiality being one of the duties owed by the fiduciary-healthcare professional), and such a duty is reinforced in the various healthcare professional codes of ethics; and there are also rights-based justifications, as patients are entitled to expect that their right to privacy (of their information) should be respected.

Confidentiality and OH Practice

We could expect confidentiality to be just as important in OH as it is in the rest of healthcare, and for the same reasons. After all, our primary purpose is protecting the health of workers, and having and maintaining their trust in OH is essential

© Springer Nature Switzerland AG 2020
J. Tamin, *Occupational Health Ethics*,
https://doi.org/10.1007/978-3-030-47283-2_4

in achieving this. But we should be mindful that there are also differences in OH practice, so I will review these differences and articulate the justifications for valuing confidentiality in OH practice.

Firstly, if we advance the reason of patient *trust* as a requirement for him to disclose relevant information for optimal *treatment* of his condition, then we may face the rebuttal that many OH professionals do not in fact *treat* patients. However, even where OH professionals are not involved in therapeutic encounters, I have suggested that we often have a *quasi-therapeutic* role (in Chap. 2). This allows us to give advice, for example, with regard workplace adjustments, safe working practices and where necessary, referrals to rehabilitation, physiotherapy or counselling. In short, it allows us to carry out our primary function, protecting worker health.

Secondly, we treat information given to us as confidential because we respect the worker's **right to privacy**. When we disclose their information, we should first obtain the worker's *permission to disclose* (rather than "informed consent", as I have argued in Chap. 3). This form of consenting recognizes the right to privacy *as well as* respecting the worker's autonomy.

Thirdly, in a fiduciary role (such as the quasi-therapeutic one), our primary loyalty is to the worker (see Chap. 2). The fiduciary obligations include a duty of confidentiality, which we must honor. However, in an *independent* role, such as when we are performing an IHR assessment, I would argue that our primary "loyalty" (or duty) is to the *commissioner* of that assessment and report (usually the pension fund manager). Even in that role, we need to treat information given to us as confidential. For example, we must not disclose information to newspapers and other media. However, I will later argue (in the section "How does this affect OH practice?"), that disclosing our findings and opinion to the commissioner of that report should **not** be considered a breach of confidentiality.

Overall, confidentiality is important in OH because we want workers, and others, to trust us. However, as I have previously mentioned (in Chap. 2), there is evidence that workers can be ambivalent about trusting OH professionals and a significant proportion mistrust us. In Chap. 2, I opined that the lack of clarity of our roles and functions could contribute to this lack of trust. In addition, in this chapter I will suggest that difficulties in understanding what confidentiality means in OH practice may be a further cause of this lack of trust. We have some specific issues in OH that we must bear in mind, such as the need to *communicate* with managers the outcome of many (probably most) of our assessments. Therefore, the problems that can arise in trying to maintain confidentiality might be more prominent in OH than in other healthcare disciplines. But before we further consider the implications of confidentiality as it pertains to OH practice, let us first remind ourselves of the difference between confidentiality and *privacy*. We will also explore the role of privacy in OH.

Privacy

Confidentiality is concerned with protecting a *relationship* of trust, as well as the *information* given within that relationship. Privacy (*informational* privacy is our interest here) is solely concerned with protecting our personal information from unauthorized access and requires **no** relationship. We are probably more accustomed to thinking about confidentiality, given that in healthcare and OH, we always have a relationship with the patient/worker. However, there may also be OH data that is collected outside this relationship, so it is important for us to be familiar with the demands of privacy, in addition to confidentiality. Moreover, although all the members of the OH team are bound by the duty of confidentiality, in this age of electronic records and data, others may have access to information originally imparted in confidence. Local arrangements will vary, but members of the information technology (IT) department, and those who might have access for audit purposes, will often be *external* to the OH department. It is essential that secure information governance procedures be in place. In these instances, it will be the worker's right to privacy, rather than confidentiality, that will protect his information.

The right to privacy is understood to be important because it gives us the space, whether physical or informational, to have the opportunity to be ourselves, and to reflect, develop and flourish. It is usually protected by national and supranational laws, such as human rights and data protection legislation.

From a worker's perspective, what is important is that he is fully aware of what happens or could happen to his information. The process should be open and transparent. He should know what information is collected and stored, and who has access to the whole or part (and if so, which part) of the information. He should be able to make corrections to the information held and alter his permissions where possible, but also be aware of what he cannot change. A privacy paradigm that allows the worker to have some control over the information held in his OH record and databases, and restricting access **only** to relevant parties (with the full knowledge of the worker) would go a long way in my view to gaining and maintaining worker trust in OH. This is hopefully the ideal we could work towards.

In the meantime, we must work within the confidentiality and privacy paradigms as they currently exist. However, there are some criticisms of the current approaches to keeping health information private and confidential, which I will explain in the next two sections.

Allowed Disclosures

Do patients or workers expect healthcare professionals to keep **all** the information they have shared, a secret? The answer probably depends on the context. A patient who needs treatment for his condition may well expect the healthcare professional to share relevant information with other members of the treating team. A worker who attends an OH consultation because his manager is asking whether he is fit to return to work will probably expect that the OH professional will need to communicate an answer back to his manager. We will consider the OH situation further in the next section. But first let us return to patients in a more general health care setting. Do patients understand what, if any, of their health information can be disclosed, to whom, and in what circumstances? There is empirical evidence that many patients are confused on this issue. It seems plausible that some of this confusion arises from the fact that there **are** instances where the healthcare professional **can** disclose information given in confidence. She may even be **required** to do so (by the courts or the regulator, for instance in the context of gun or knife injuries). Some ethicists have criticized this form of confidentiality. They argue that permitting or requiring such disclosures could lead to *mistrust* of healthcare professionals, rather than trust. Although I believe that they make valid points, we have to work within the current confidentiality paradigm, imperfect as it may be. We can try to achieve better patient trust by being very open and transparent about the instances where we might need to breach confidentiality. They should understand the limits of confidentiality and the reasons why we might need to breach it, preferably even before the consultation (for example, in correspondence with the appointment details). We should then reinforce pertinent parts of this message before and during the consultation, where this is appropriate.

So, when can we disclose patient information? Disclosures are allowed (i) if the patient consents; (ii) if the disclosure is required by law; or (iii), if it is in the public interest.

When a patient does give consent (or *permission*, see Chap. 3) for us to disclose of some of his information, then such a disclosure should not put at risk the trust he has in healthcare professionals. However, we must still be careful that his permission has been given voluntarily, and that he knows to whom the disclosure will be made, and he understands the purpose of that disclosure. As long as these requirements are met, then this type of allowed disclosure is being made in an open and transparent manner. I do not think that patients would feel that their trust in the healthcare professional had been breached with this type of disclosure.

The second type of allowed disclosure, that is, when it is required by law, will vary according to national and regional laws, so I will not address this in depth here. However, I would emphasize that we **must** follow our national laws. We should also note that this disclosure would be *without* the patient's permission. We may therefore feel in a legal-ethical double bind. There are no easy solutions to the conflict we may feel in such circumstances. However, as long as it is safe for us to do so, we should inform the patient of the situation, and ensure that disclosure is **only** to parties that are entitled to the information.

The third type of allowed disclosure is when this is *in the public interest*. This is usually justified on the basis that **not** disclosing this information would put a third party or third parties at risk of harm, so the principle of non-maleficence comes into play. However, we have seen previously that there is also a public (as well as private) interest in *maintaining* confidentiality (that is, to promote public trust in healthcare professionals). Therefore, these conflicting interests need to be balanced against each other, and this is can be difficult. For example, if there were a significant risk of death or serious injury from non-disclosure, then we can feel justified in breaching confidentiality. But what if the injury is less serious, or less likely to occur? As OH professionals, we are used to the concept and practice of risk assessments, and this is what is required here. However, there is usually still a degree of subjectivity involved in assessing risk in this way, so we may not always feel comfortable with our decision. It would be prudent to discuss such difficult scenarios with experienced colleagues, and maybe use an ethical reflective tool (for example, see Appendix 4) to help with this discussion.

Indeed, we could argue that in OH, we are more often involved in situations where disclosure "in the public interest" are likely to occur, given that we deal with workers in safety critical roles. We will therefore explore in greater depth how the allowed disclosures could and do affect OH practice.

How Does This Affect OH Practice?

Earlier in this chapter, we discussed the importance of confidentiality itself in OH practice. Here, I will specifically look at the effect of *allowed disclosures* on OH practice.

I believe there are three main reasons why allowed breaches may have greater (or at least more noticeable) impact on OH practice, compared with the rest of healthcare. Firstly, the **output** of most (probably virtually all) OH consultations and assessments usually consists of some *communication* to the employer. Secondly, our *dual obligations* make our duty to third parties more explicit. Thirdly, as I mentioned above, many of us will look after workers in safety critical roles. Thus, disclosures *in the public interest* may arise more frequently in our practice.

In addition, the legal position in some countries is that an OH professional disclosing information pertaining to an assessment, when the purpose of that assessment relates to fitness for work, does **not** breach the duty of confidentiality. This clearly goes *beyond* the allowed disclosures listed above. From a legal perspective, one of the leading cases cited in the context of OH confidentiality is the US case of *Bratt* versus *IBM*. The courts held that the employer had a legitimate business interest in having the medical information which their company doctor passed to managers: "when medical information is necessary reasonably to serve such a substantial and valid interest of the employer, it is not an invasion of privacy, for a physician to disclose such information to the employer." Although I have also cited UK case law, as well as several ethical commentaries (including one from me) in the "Notes" to this chapter, which all support the view that an OH professional does not breach confidentiality when disclosing relevant information to the employer, this "additional" allowed disclosure does require further qualification and elaboration.

The first important qualification is that the worker must have consented to the assessment *process* and understood that the results of that assessment will usually be communicated to the employer. This is the informed consent (IC) part of the consenting process (see Chap. 3) and applies to **all** OH assessments. Moreover, if the OH professional is in a quasi-therapeutic relationship with the worker for this assessment (see Chap. 2), then the worker's permission is further required before the information is sent to the employer (the exception being in cases of risk of harm to third parties). If the OH professional is in an independent role (such as for ill-health retirement assessments), *further* permission to disclose the report may not be required (this is the position I support, but some colleagues may disagree). However, in all cases the OH professional should make it clear to the worker what information will be relayed and to whom. In addition, the OH professional should avoid disclosing unnecessarily sensitive and personal information. I prefer to avoid disclosing clinical details unless these are essential. It is usually sufficient for the employer to understand the implications relating to the worker's fitness for work and/or work adjustments in *functional terms*, for example, what type of work activity needs to be avoided or what needs to be modified. I will illustrate how this can be done in practice in Chap. 6 ("Report writing").

To summarize, although we have legal and ethical support for the view that our communications to employers do not usually constitute a breach of confidence, we should still proceed with caution. If we communicate worker information in ways that make them distrust us, then we will have done a serious disservice to OH as a whole. We must be honest and transparent in how and what we communicate to employers and obtain workers' permission to disclose their information where appropriate. If workers are unsure about how we maintain confidentiality, then this will reduce the likelihood of them trusting us. In addition, when we consider the different roles and functions (which affect our fiduciary duties) that we undertake (see Chap. 2), then it can make confidentiality in OH practice very difficult to understand. So, it is not surprising that patients and workers become confused about what information they can entrust to the OH professional, and when that confidentiality might be (legally and ethically) breached.

Chapter 6 ("Report writing") is about all types of OH communications (mainly to the employer). This will give us the opportunity to see how the current (and sometimes conflicting, such as the "allowed disclosures") confidentiality paradigm might work in our OH practice, especially by means of the *case vignettes* in the "Management referral reports" section. You will later see from those examples how important I believe it is to work *with* workers and to involve them in their difficult ethical situations when these arise, before we communicate with the employer. By working through these various scenarios, I hope that it will become clearer to you what I believe confidentiality means or should mean in our day to day OH practice. As we gain a better understanding of OH confidentiality, then we can make this clearer also for our patients, the workers, employers and others we interact with.

Conclusion

Confidentiality is crucially important in OH practice, as it is in the rest of healthcare.

Workers have a right to expect us to respect the privacy of their information. Moreover, we owe workers a duty of confidentiality, which aims to protect both their information and the relationship of trust within which this information is shared. The privacy and confidentiality of OH *records* and worker health data are reasonably straightforward: these should be accessible only by the OH team. There is no difference to the rest of healthcare in this aspect.

Unfortunately, the difficult legal and ethical rules around confidentiality, especially when it may be breached (to prevent third party harm for example), may contribute to some mistrust in healthcare and OH professionals, instead of the trust it is intended to foster. This is arguably even more confusing in OH, where we need to communicate some worker information to employers (for example through *reports* that we write) as part of our daily practice. However, if we can be clearer ourselves about what these rules are, then we can explain these more clearly to workers and employers. This could go a long way to restoring and improving trust in OH, which is important if we want to protect worker health effectively.

Chapter 5
Sickness Absence

Introduction

In some countries, OH professionals deal with referrals (by management) of workers who are "off sick" as a major proportion of their work. In other countries, such as Belgium, OH professionals are not involved with the sickness absence of workers, and this topic would be covered by "insurance medicine". However, whether sickness absence is covered by OH or insurance medicine, the subject of ill-health and inability to work is an important one in many ways, as we will see later. But you may wonder why the topic of "sickness absence", which could be viewed as a very practical topic, as it is one that we encounter on a day-to-day basis, should be in this "theory" section of the book. The reason for this is that I would like to address the ethical issues that arise out of the relationship between inability to work and ill-health in a *broader* sense here. This will call for an understanding of theories of and approaches to social justice, so these theories will be introduced in this chapter.

Although our main focus will be on fairness and equity in the context of 'long term' sickness absence (often taken to mean longer than four weeks), I will also include a short commentary on the fairness of some aspects of HR absence or "attendance" policies (which will relate mainly to 'short term' sickness absence) at the end of this chapter.

Health, Work and the Disadvantaged

In some countries, sickness absence is said to be a huge financial burden to the state. For example, it is reported to cost the UK economy £100 billion a year. One of the suggested solutions in the UK is for access to OH services to be increased. Our role would be to give advice in the context of *sickness absence management*, which for many OH professionals is one of our main activities anyway (albeit this does not apply to all countries, as noted above). Sickness absence management does bring to the

© Springer Nature Switzerland AG 2020
J. Tamin, *Occupational Health Ethics*,
https://doi.org/10.1007/978-3-030-47283-2_5

fore some of the conflicts of interest and ethical tension between workers, employers and us. For example, we must balance our duty to protect the confidentiality of worker information against our duty to give the employer information relevant to their needs, such as information which enables them to discharge their health and safety obligations, or to run their business. I will discuss such types of ethical conflicts later in Chap. 6 (Report writing), especially in the "Management referral reports" section. As I have mentioned earlier, here I would like to look *beyond* our role of giving advice in such situations. I believe that OH has an important and unique role to play in the ethical issues that arise out of health and work. I think ICOH also echoes this belief when it exhorts us to act on "the principle of equity" to assist workers in obtaining and maintaining employment notwithstanding their health impairments or disabilities.

In an ICOH report (2017), it is mentioned that OH professionals are in a *key position* to provide the preventive, protective and individually adjusted services that the different groups of **vulnerable** workers need. Workers can be more vulnerable because of: (i) their economic and social circumstances; (ii) being in high risk occupations; or (iii) their health or psycho-physiological situation. Moreover, when we consider the strong links between poverty, lower education attainment, unemployment (or less favorable employment) and poor health (often described as the "social determinants of health"), then it is likely that there is considerable overlap between the groups of vulnerable workers. For example, someone who is poor and has little education may feel more compelled to accept an insecure job, as he is desperate to earn some income, and each of these factors (that is, poverty, lower educational attainment and job insecurity) are independently linked to poorer health. In turn impaired health can also make it more difficult to find good employment (although hopefully OH can have a positive influence on this). Therefore, the different types of disadvantage (social, economic, educational, employment and health) can **compound** each other in multi-dimensional ways. Given that there are an estimated 1.5 billion vulnerable workers globally (ICOH 2017, p. 14), this is a significant challenge for all countries, and we as OH professionals can have an important role in addressing this.

We know that **good** work is good for health. Good work tends to have the following characteristics: it is work for which we feel we are suitably recompensed; we feel that we are treated fairly; we have some control over the way we work; and we can develop and progress at work. Participation in this type of work is so much *more* than just having an income. It can help give us a sense of purpose, improve our self-worth and social inclusion. There are so many multi-layered ways it can improve our physical and psychological health. The converse is also true: *bad* work (such as insecure jobs) can seriously damage our health. **Bad work can be just as bad for health as being unemployed** (see WHO 2003 reference 8 in Notes), and unemployment causes more illness and premature death! As OH professionals, I believe we should constantly remind employers and policy makers of this important relationship between work and health. This health-work relationship applies to all workers, but some groups of vulnerable workers are at greater risk of being in lower paid jobs and being treated less favorably. One such group of vulnerable workers includes those who are disabled, and we will consider the relationship between disability, health and work in the next section.

Disability

There are various conceptions and definitions of disability. These range from a focus on the individual's impairments or conditions (the "medical model" of disability) on the one hand, to an emphasis on the social configurations and arrangements which can either be functionally limiting or enabling to the individual (the "social model") on the other. To my mind, a combination of both approaches is probably the most helpful for our purposes. An example of this is the UNCRPD definition, which notes *both* the individual impairments, whether physical, psychological, intellectual or sensory, **and** the barriers which may "hinder their full and effective participation in society on an equal basis with others". As OH professionals, we are very familiar with this in practice. One of our major contributions in this area is to advise on adjustments to the working environment and/or conditions which can enable those with impairments to function successfully in a wider number of jobs. Without such support and modifications in the workplace, those with impairments might otherwise have struggled in some of these jobs or have been deemed "unfit" for such work. Thus, we have much first-hand experience of how altering the social (in this case, work) environment and support can make such a difference to a disabled individual's ability to fully and effectively participate "in society on an equal basis with others".

Of course, not all disabled individuals are poor, and some may not consider themselves to have a health problem. Indeed, Paralympians are elite athletes who would outperform most of us in many ways! But many disabled people are trapped in "multidimensional poverty". The multiple dimensions that compound their poverty include poor health, lower educational attainment and less favorable (or no) employment. For example, one can understand that someone with a long-term health impairment might miss a lot of schooling and not be able to achieve good educational qualifications. This in turn limits their options in the job market. Lower income might make it more difficult to afford treatment for their condition, participate in social activities and afford better quality food, which in turn all cause their health to deteriorate further. In addition, it has been noted that the disabled have greater difficulty in converting earnings into improvements in their quality of life (called a "conversion handicap") because of the additional costs of overcoming the disadvantages of their disability. For example, if they have mobility problems, then it may cost them more to travel. In a study of disabled households in the UK, it was concluded that this conversion handicap is around 30-40%, depending on which metric is being considered.

One of the ways out of this poverty trap can be through paid employment. Furthermore, if we take account of the beneficial effects of good work (as mentioned previously), then there is even greater reason to facilitate the employment of disadvantaged disabled individuals. So, OH can play an important role in alleviating this otherwise depressing picture. But we should also note that the description of "vulnerable workers" in the ICOH 2017 report (as mentioned in the previous section) is apposite for the disadvantaged disabled workers in *all* three domains: the disabled can be more vulnerable on socio-economic grounds, on health grounds, *and* they may also be in less good (and riskier) jobs. Therefore, the role of OH professionals in providing "preventive, protective and individually adjusted services" for this group of disadvantaged and vulnerable workers is *especially* important. What do I mean by this? To explain our role here, or the role I believe we should have, let us consider the following two areas of interest:

(i)   Firstly, what is the reported experience of disabled workers at work? Unfortunately, an in-depth study of disabled workers in the UK suggests that a significant number of them are treated unfairly, discriminated against (in spite of legislation designed to prevent this), and even humiliated in their workplaces. We know that such *bad* work is as damaging to health as unemployment.

(ii) Secondly, we know that **good** work is good for health. Therefore, accessing such good work would give the disadvantaged disabled an opportunity to improve their health, as well as their income. As OH professionals carrying out pre-employment assessments (and later, sickness absence assessments), we are well placed to advise against any unnecessary barriers to them obtaining (and then retaining) such work.

Therefore, much of OH practice can be of direct benefit to disabled individuals (and one can argue that this benefits society as a whole). For example, we know how to make individual assessments and recommend appropriate workplace adjustments. We know when to recommend individual risk assessments to prevent harm to the health of a worker with a specific vulnerability. So much of our expertise in the field of OH can help remove unnecessary barriers and prejudices when advising on the suitability of disabled individuals to work.

Moreover, as OH professionals, we are uniquely placed at the health-work interface, and I believe we have an equitable duty to share our insights and experiences to **influence** employers and policy makers (whether employer or State policies) to help the disadvantaged and vulnerable workers (and those of working age) in matters of work and health. To help us frame our arguments for fairer and more supportive workplaces, I believe it would help us to have some general understanding of how the ethics of justice and fairness is discussed and argued. In the next two sections, we will firstly explore some of the theories of and approaches to social justice; and secondly consider the *capability approach* in greater depth.

Theories of Justice

If we are interested in living in a just society, on what basis could we or should we determine what is just or unjust, fair or unfair? In order to answer this question, let us briefly review some of the prevailing schools of thought on this subject.

In the last few decades, the dominant theoretical conception of justice has been based on that advanced by John Rawls. His formulation of an *egalitarian* theory of justice has markedly influenced policy in many spheres, ranging from political philosophy to welfare economics. Although Rawls himself did not apply his theory of justice to health and health care, others such as Norman Daniels, have extended the Rawlsian approach to critically analyze whether health policies were just and fair, for example. The egalitarian theories emphasize the importance of **equal** access to goods and opportunities (although some inequalities can be justified under certain conditions). This conceptual basis for a just society differs from another important theoretical approach, namely the *utilitarian* theories of justice, which emphasize the need to maximize social utility. Rights and obligations are understood in the light of achieving this end.

Although the main theories of justice can sometimes be seen as conflicting with one another, it is also possible to take a pluralistic approach, drawing on the salient features of one or other to understand and analyze a particular problem or context. Alternatively, some theories have been developed for a specific context. An example of this would be the *well-being* theories, which stress the right to health, and argue that justice involves reducing health inequalities.

In the context that is of interest to us here, namely that of disadvantaged and vulnerable populations, a new approach seems to be particularly apt. This is the *capability* approach, which we will consider in greater detail in the next section.

The Capability Approach

In this section, I will argue that the capability approach (CA) provides us with the most useful theoretical framework in conceptualizing social justice and the ethical issues around our OH role in relation to disadvantaged vulnerable workers.

This approach to social justice was first articulated by Amartya Sen, Nobel Prize laureate in Economics. Its focus is on the individual: what she is able **to be** and what she is able **to do** (her "capabilities"); and what she actually achieves in terms of beings and doings (her "functionings"). The role of a fair social system or structure is to enable her to achieve her capabilities. But whether she converts these into functionings is up to her, as the CA holds the notion of *agency* (or her right to make choices in the light of her values) as pivotal. Martha Nussbaum, a philosopher, has been very influential in the development of the CA and she particularly highlights the importance of respect for *human dignity* in this approach. She also specified ten "central capabilities", whereas Sen did not specify the capabilities, advising instead that different communities could agree through public debate and reasoning, which ones mattered most in their context.

We may already be familiar with one practical application of the CA, in the form of the United Nations Human Development Index (HDI), which has been used for example, to correlate OH services coverage with countries according to their HDI, in an ICOH survey of Global OHS coverage. The HDI offers an alternative metric to the GNP (Gross National Product) in welfare economics and is more relevant to our interest in the welfare of individuals, especially of vulnerable workers and disadvantaged groups.

An exciting new development in the fields of OH and the CA has been the pioneering work by researchers based at Tilburg University and other institutions, under the leadership of Professor van der Klink. They have developed firstly a conceptual model of sustainable working life based on the CA, and secondly a "Working Role Functioning Questionnaire" (WRFQ), also based on the CA. This approach considers work capability to be present if a worker values a particular aspect of her work, and the work arrangements allow her to achieve this value herself. This focus on what workers value in their work and enabling them to achieve these particular functionings makes it so much more likely that their work will be "good work". It places the worker's agency and having opportunities to flourish in her job at the very **centre** of their evaluation. This work capability paradigm would be of benefit to *all* workers, but this approach may be especially protective of *vulnerable* workers' health and wellbeing (such as protecting them from the negative experiences at work that I previously mentioned in relation to disabled workers).

Unfair Policies?

Let us now return to the topic of sickness absence more generally. In particular, let us consider the HR policies that our organizations use to regulate sickness absence, which may be called an "Absence Policy" or an "Attendance Policy", for example. I would like to review aspects which I consider to be unfair in these policies and see whether the insights drawn from social justice and fairness (as discussed above), help us with this review.

Do we have any legitimate interest in whether HR policies are fair and just? Well, ICOH in its Code of Ethics does advise us that the organizations that employ us should have "a programme of organizational ethics that is aligned with the ethical principles" of the Code, that is, *our* ethical principles. Those principles, listed in our Code, include the principle of equity and respect for human dignity. I believed that we are justified therefore, in seeking values such as fairness and respect for human dignity in HR and other organizational policies. For my critiques of these policies, I will use two examples: The first will be Elsie's case (from the Prologue of this book); the second will be the situation of Health Care Workers (HCWs) with a transient transmissible infection, such as an influenza-like illness or a gastro-intestinal infection.

Elsie

What Elsie and her family experienced towards the end of her life was a real tragedy and to my mind, an example of HR bureaucracy "gone mad". Here I must pause. It has been suggested that we should take account of personal, professional and institutional ethics to resolve ethical conflicts. I fully concur with this. I also accept that organizations have a legitimate reason to have policies that maximize worker attendance, increase productivity and reduce costs. But I must admit that my personal and professional ethics get the better of me. I think that sacking Elsie after so many years of loyal service, at the time when she was at her most vulnerable, should seem unjust to *any* reasonable person. Also, if we are not compassionate and believe in upholding human dignity, then we would not be doing the job we are in, as OH professionals.

Is there a more objective and less emotive way to look at Elsie's case? Well, I think we are looking for an approach in HR policies that would ensure some fairness in the way Elsie was treated at that point. Ironically, in the UK, disability legislation is well developed but it still did not protect Elsie. The HR manager probably acted within the law in applying the Attendance Policy so rigidly. This is in line with Fevre's comment (see in the "Disability" section) that the disabled were not adequately protected at work, notwithstanding existing legislation. So, would moral theories of justice help Elsie? I have commended the CA as being the most helpful in our context of OH and vulnerable workers. However, using the WRFQ would not have alerted us to any problem, as Elsie was in a job where she felt valued and she could achieve her work capabilities while she was healthy. It is more at a conceptual level that the CA could have made a difference. When the HR Attendance Policy was written, if values that the CA holds central (albeit other theories of justice may also hold one or more as important), such as respect for human dignity, agency, and opportunities for the individual to attain valuable functionings, had been considered, then I believe Elsie would have been better treated by the organization.

Health Care Workers

Let us now turn to another situation where I believe HR Attendance Policies can be unfair, namely that which arises when health care workers (HCWs) develop an infective illness, such as an influenza-type one or gastro-enteritis (typically causing diarrhoea and vomiting). Because of the risk of transmission to patients, Infection Control Policies require them to stay off work until they are deemed not to present an infection risk to patients. This seems sensible and appropriate. However, it usually means that they fall foul of HR Attendance Policies for "repeated short-term sickness absence", with consequent penalties, such as staged warnings that can eventually lead to dismissal. In the UK hospitals I am familiar with, there is **no** allowance made for the fact that another policy (that is, for infection control) **requires** them to stay off work!

So, what is the HCW to do? Should she ignore the risk to patients, and attend work anyway? Surely, her professional (and personal) ethics would prevent her from putting patients at risk if she is still infectious. But staying away from work puts her at risk of being dismissed, thereby incurring financial harm to herself and her family. She finds herself in an ethical double bind situation. Is it fair that the organization puts HCWs in such a position? I think the unfairness of the Health Care organizations' position is patently obvious to everyone, and one does not have to appeal to any specific theory of justice to demonstrate this unfairness. However, I would suggest that if the organizations truly valued their staff as individuals worthy of respect, then they would not put them in this impossible situation.

Here, my aim is to raise the ethical point rather than to offer any definite solutions. I would suggest that it would be for the hospital management and staff representatives to discuss this double bind situation, and work towards a policy that would be fair to the staff and safe for their patients, in their specific context.

Conclusion

In this chapter on sickness absence, we have discussed the plight of vulnerable workers and the key roles that OH professionals can play in this context. In particular, we have considered the situation of disabled workers, who can be vulnerable in more ways than one. We noted that some employers' approaches to sickness absence could be disproportionately unfair to disabled workers. I described the capability approach (CA) as my favoured approach to justice and fairness in our OH context. The central roles that agency and human dignity play in the CA are especially valuable when we want to prevent behaviours at work that devalue and belittle individuals. Our primary purpose is to protect the health of workers at work and to promote healthy behaviours. It then follows that we should act and advise against organizational practices that allow bullying, discrimination and unfair practices. We should do this both at *practitioner level*, for example, giving unbiased and evidence-based advice to both workers and managers; and at *policy level*, for those of us who are in a position where we can influence organizational policies, we should advise that these policies must be fair and equitable. Fairness is health enhancing.

Part II
Practice

Chapter 6
Report Writing

In this chapter, and in subsequent chapters, we move from exploring the theoretical basis of our moral reasoning and decision-making, to applying these theories and approaches to our day-to-day OH *practice*.

As OH professionals, we need to communicate with parties *other than* the workers (our "patients") on a regular basis. This communication is often in the form of a written report. It is therefore apposite to start our practical section with the topic of *report writing*, as this is an activity we frequently perform, and one that brings together much of the theoretical ethics we have previously discussed. For example, we should consider ethical issues such as whether we have the worker's *permission to disclose* (Chap. 3), and whether we are observing the rules of *confidentiality* (Chap. 4) when we are writing and transmitting our report. We also should be mindful of which of the *OH roles* (Chap. 2) we are performing at the time, as this will vary depending on the context and purpose of our assessment and subsequent report. We will begin our exploration of such ethical issues with the pre-employment assessment report.

Pre-employment Assessment Reports

Pre-employment assessments, also sometimes known as pre-placement assessments, are a standard feature of OH practice. Although my focus in this section is on the *report* that we write and send to the employer after this assessment, some of the ethical issues that arise in writing the report are linked to the *assessment* itself. For example, ethical tension may arise when we conclude that the proposed job may place the applicant at increased risk of harm to his health. It would then require us to balance our primary goal of protecting the *health* of the worker from against the need to respect his *autonomy*, should he decide that he would rather take that risk, because he needs the income from that job. The ethical tensions then might manifest themselves in terms of the report we need to communicate to the employer, but those tensions only arise because the worker is not happy with the advice we are proposing to communicate. We will return to such conflicting ethical demands later

© Springer Nature Switzerland AG 2020
J. Tamin, *Occupational Health Ethics*,
https://doi.org/10.1007/978-3-030-47283-2_6

in this section and explore ways to address these. But before we do so, let us reflect on some of the ethical issues that a pre-employment assessment *itself* may raise.

Firstly, the pre-employment assessment should *not* be used to reject applicants on the basis of their health or disability, if they have the necessary qualifications etc. for the job and would be able to do this job. Therefore, we should only assess those who have received a *firm* offer for the job (possibly with a "subject to medical" proviso), so that suitable applicants are not subjected to unfair disability discrimination. Secondly, there is some evidence that *routine* pre-employment assessments may be of little value, so it raises the question as to whether it is ethical (if it is of little benefit) to carry out such activity in the first place (especially if resources are limited or the assessment is invasive). This is especially likely to be the case in low risk occupations, such as administrative posts. However, there should still be the option to assess where it would be of benefit, for example, for an OH professional to be able to recommend workplace adjustments for someone with a disability or chronic health condition; or a specific risk assessment for an applicant with an increased vulnerability to some workplace exposure (such as to psychosocial pressures). Thirdly, this assessment should not be unnecessarily discriminatory. By this, I mean that any medical standards applied should be justifiable, and **evidence-based** as much as possible. Additionally, any questions, examinations, or investigations must not be unduly intrusive. Once again, they need to be evidence-based, and relate directly to fitness to perform the intended job (including third party safety), or to the workplace hazards (so as to protect the applicant's health). I think it also essential that the OH professionals advising on such matters, both in setting up the assessment process, and in carrying out the individual assessments, should be **competent** (that is, have appropriate OH training and expertise) and have good knowledge (preferably first hand) of the workplace and its hazards. Lastly, there should be an appeal process for applicants who wish to challenge the OH professional's advice. The establishment of such an appeals procedure should help to promote worker (or applicant) trust that the system is designed to be fair.

Let us now turn to the report itself. The *purpose* of this report is to advise the employer whether the applicant is medically fit for this job, whether he requires any adjustments to the job or work environment, and whether he requires additional risk assessments because of some specific vulnerabilities. Our *role* here is as an independent adviser (see Chap. 2). We maintain *confidentiality* by only disclosing relevant (and limited, see below) information to the relevant party or parties (such as his manager and/or an HR professional). We need to explain all this to the applicant at the start of the process so that he can give *informed consent* to the assessment, and *permission to disclose* the subsequent report.

We have a duty to advise the employer, as this is usually the way we will be able to protect the health of the prospective worker (and other workers) in this work environment. In addition, we may have a contractual duty to inform the employer of the applicant's fitness status. However, we also owe a duty of confidentiality to this prospective worker. These ethical duties may sometimes be in conflict. We can reduce this conflict in the following ways:

Firstly, the processes of obtaining informed consent (IC) to do the assessment, and permission to disclose (PTD) the subsequent report require us to have explained the *purpose* of this pre-employment assessment, as I mentioned above. At this stage, we should ensure that the applicant has fully understood this. Most applicants will have the capacity to understand, but we need to use language that is accessible to them. On this note, if we believe that the applicant may lack capacity to understand this information, then we must ensure that the appropriate arrangements are in place (see "Capacity" in Chap. 3).

Secondly, the IC and particularly the PTD processes should make clear to the applicant *who* will be receiving this report (usually the relevant manager and the Human Resources Department), *what* information it might contain and for what *reasons*. In my practice, I like to explain that I do not routinely give clinical diagnoses or other clinical information in my reports. The report would usually confirm fitness or not to do the job (with or without restrictions), and whether I advise any adjustments or additional risk assessments. It focusses on the **functional** implications of any condition(s), rather than the condition(s) itself or themselves. For example, I think it is more important for a manager to know that a worker could have episodes of loss of awareness, rather than being told that this new worker has a diagnosis of "petit mal epilepsy". This avoids unnecessary stigmatization, and maybe even discrimination. As we know, most conditions have wide variability, and it is how the **individual** is affected that matters. If the condition is well controlled on medication, and episodes are very infrequent, then there may be the need for very little in the way of adjustments. As with all conditions, it is important for us to consider whether timing of medications, shifts and long hours, and other work factors or patterns, could affect the condition, and if so, give advice on these factors. If there is a safety element to the job, then an in-depth risk assessment is needed. We should give input into this risk assessment, such as the likelihood of occurrence (we may need more information from the applicant's GP or neurologist), how much warning he has (such as "aura"), and what actions his colleagues and manager should take in the event of an episode. We should also advise specifically (if these are features of the job) on lone working, working at heights, driving at work, and any other relevant safety at work considerations. The applicant should understand that this is the type of advice we would give in a report, and the employer should also understand that this is the type of information a report to them would contain, rather than any *clinical* information.

However, there are occasions when giving *some* clinical information may be helpful for both the prospective worker and the employer. It is still important to gain the applicant's permission to disclose this, and they must be aware of what (limited) clinical information is being disclosed. For example, in the case of an applicant with insulin dependent diabetes, although it is possible to make the adjustments and risk assessment recommendations without disclosing the diagnosis, I find that most applicants are happy for the diagnosis to be disclosed. This would still be on a "need to know" basis, such as the manager, supervisors and first aiders, for example. The further information relating to this diagnosis should be limited to whatever is relevant to protect the applicant's health (such as attending specialist review appointments), or the safety of the public (for example, in the case of healthcare workers or drivers).

Much of the useful advice is in the form of non-clinical information, for example adjustments may include offering prompt access to their sugary drinks or snacks if they feel they are becoming hypoglycemic; and the availability if required of a clean (and private) area to inject their insulin and test their blood sugar levels.

By limiting the information to what is strictly needed for employers to know, it is more likely that worker trust in OH professionals and OH services will be maintained. I also believe that by so doing, we can achieve the dual purpose of protecting the prospective worker's health (by sharing appropriate information with the employer) *and* respecting the individual's right to confidentiality and privacy (as the worker is usually happy about giving permission to disclose the relevant information).

I think this approach generally serves us well for most of our pre-employment assessments and reports. However, problems still do arise on occasions. Let us consider two specific such instances: the first is when the applicant has been found unfit for the job and is not happy with this outcome; the second is when the applicant refuses to give his permission for disclosure of the report.

The first scenario (of an applicant being found "unfit") is relatively rare in practice. This is because our emphasis should be on specifying in our advice to the employer what restrictions, adjustments and additional risk assessments *might* make the applicant fit for the job. It would then be the employer's decision as to whether they can accommodate these restrictions and adjustments, and whether they consider the extra cost of putting these in place reasonable. There are occasions however, when the applicant does not meet a statutory (or other regulatory) medical standard and so is medically not fit for the job (regardless of adjustments). On other occasions, it may be that they have poor insight into, or have poor control of, their condition. I think that it is often their lack of insight or their poor control rather than the condition *itself*, that makes them unfit for the job *at that time* (arguably, both could be improved with the right therapeutic approaches). This is especially relevant where others, such as other workers or members of the public (such as patients), could be put at risk if the applicant did not have good control of their condition and/or lacked insight. The conditions could be physical such as insulin dependent diabetes, or psychiatric, such as a psychotic illness. These are usually difficult consultations, specially if the applicant has poor insight. They may challenge your advice on their fitness for the job. This is when it is particularly helpful to be able to point them to an appeal procedure that they can access. Arrangements for such an appeal process will vary depending on your organization, but I often find that offering access to an independent OH professional outside the organization (as long as they are familiar with safety etc. requirements of the job and your organization) for a "second opinion" defuses the situation. So, having an appeal process demonstrates not only fairness for the applicant, it can also take some of the pressure off the OH professional in these circumstances.

The second scenario, namely when the applicant refuses to give his permission for the report to be disclosed, could arise as a result of his being found unfit for the job. It may also arise when the applicant, although deemed medically fit for the job, is not happy with the information you propose to disclose in the report. In either situation, the lack of a report (or "fitness certificate") would usually mean that the applicant will not be able to be employed in that job. This is different to the ill-health retirement situation, as I will explain later. So, it is possible to take the view that it is the applicant's choice, that he understands the consequences of his refusal, and to simply record the refusal in his OH notes. It could be debated whether we could inform the employer that we had not received permission to disclose the fitness report without further permission! In this situation (that is, the pre-employment one), it probably does not matter much in practice, as the employer should take it that without a fitness certificate, the applicant is not able to start the job. However, you may feel that this is a rather unsatisfactory state of affairs, and I would agree. I do not believe there to be a strong ethical argument to favor one approach over the other, although it could be argued that trust in OH services would be enhanced if we tried to resolve problems when they occur. So, in the case where the applicant is found to be unfit, I would encourage him to allow this to be disclosed, but to use the appeal procedure. In the case where he *is* fit but does not like the information that the report is disclosing, I would happily review this with him. Is there terminology that seems too value-laden? Too clinical? Is there a way of giving the advice in more *functional* terms, and achieving the same result? Or if there is disagreement over the extent of adjustments, for example, could an acceptable compromise be found? As a last resort, the appeal procedure may also help in this scenario.

Some might question the validity of the consenting processes (both, informed consent (IC) for the assessment and permission to disclose (PTD) the report) if refusal of either IC or PTD, or both, would inevitably lead to the applicant *not* being offered the job. To expand on this line of argument, in Chap. 3, we recognized that for consent to be valid, it must be **freely** given, and there should be no coercion involved, otherwise this would not constitute true consent. However, in the pre-employment situation, if the applicant does not comply with the process, he is usually not employed. So, is there some degree of coercion? One response to this could be that he is free to apply or not for this job. The opposite view would be that, if he is desperate to get this job, he may agree to anything, but it would not truly reflect free choice. I believe there is some validity in both positions. On the one hand, many choices we make in life are not completely "free", but we (individually and as communities) *do* make these choices nonetheless. That is, we may be prepared to trade off some of our freedom or autonomy in order to achieve something else that we value, such as adhering to speed limits and traffic signals to make our roads safer; or tolerating the relative invasion of privacy from security cameras in our town centers to lessen the threat of violence. On the other hand, an applicant in this position could be in a particularly vulnerable position, so I believe that as OH professionals, we have a responsibility to ensure that the pre-employment assessment is as fair, non-discriminatory and evidence-based as possible. For example, we should resist attempts from an employer to perform unnecessary and intrusive investigations, such as HIV or genetic testing, unless the job required such testing on regulatory or evidence-based grounds.

Management Referral Reports

By management referral (MR) reports, I mean reports (in any form, whether paper or electronic) that we write to managers (and/or HR) following our assessment of a worker referred to us by the employer (usually the manager or HR). This will usually arise during the course of the worker's employment, but also sometimes after their employment (such as for "deferred" pension cases, that is, those ex-workers who apply for early release of their pension on health grounds). We will consider the latter situation in the next section ("Ill-health retirement reports").

A manager may refer a worker to the OH department for a multitude of reasons. These range from questions about a worker's ongoing fitness for work; questions as to whether performance problems might be a result of health problems; or questions regarding the reasons and duration of any time taken off work attributed to ill-health (sickness absence, which may come under "insurance medicine" in some countries, see Chap. 5). In addition, sometimes the employer will ask about the fitness of a worker to attend a disciplinary hearing; or may refer because of concerns about a worker's behavior at work; and so on. MR reports therefore cover a wide spectrum of OH practice, and thus can also reflect the range of ethical tensions and conflicts that we face in our day to day work.

This type of assessment and report gives us good opportunities to examine the application of our moral approaches in real life OH situations. I will try to replicate some of the issues we face in our OH practice, by first describing four case vignettes, which I have chosen because they can be particularly challenging and problematic for different reasons. After I have described these vignettes, we will explore the ethical concerns each of them may raise.

Case Vignettes

i.   Lorraine is a teacher of more than 20 years' experience. Her headteacher referred her to the OH department because of repeated episodes of sickness absence in the last year. The "fit notes" issued by her GP (general practitioner, or family doctor) have given different reasons for absence at various times, including gastroenteritis, influenza and stress. In his referral letter, the head mentions that Lorraine looks after her mother, who suffers from dementia, and he states that he is "concerned about her wellbeing". In a previous meeting with the head, you recall that he "does not believe in stress".

When you meet Lorraine, she comes across as a dedicated teacher, who loves her work. In the last year, her mother's health has deteriorated and this has been a source of worry to her. However, she attributes most of her stress to changes at work. There have been staff shortages, and she has had to stay late most evenings to keep up with her work demands. She also brings a lot of work home which she does at night and weekends. In addition, she has been given the responsibility for Health & Safety for the whole school just a month ago, although she has no prior experience in this field. The previous incumbent had resigned. There will be an external inspection within the next few weeks, and she is worried about the state of the paperwork, such as the Health & Safety policy and risk assessments. She tried to approach the head with her work concerns, but he was dismissive with "well, we are all busy". She has not been sleeping well. She realizes that she is short-tempered with her family at home and feels guilty about this. She has had problems with her concentration both at work and at home, for example, she would find herself reading the same page several times, which was unusual for her. Her GP has suggested anti-depressants and counselling, but she has not taken up his offer of either so far. She does not feel counselling would help her as this would not resolve the problems she faces arising from work.

ii. Ashley is a staff nurse whose ward manager is concerned about his possible alcohol misuse, but she has not mentioned this to him. However, she writes in her OH referral letter that he has triggered the absence policy with 3 episodes of sickness absence and would like him to "have a check-up" to rule out any underlying health condition (the stated diagnoses on the self-certificates were: sprained ankle, diarrhea and back pain). She does not mention alcohol in her letter but had an "off the record" conversation with your OH manager. She mentioned that colleagues had cited instances where Ashley had had slurred speech and they thought they could smell alcohol on his breath. There had been no patient complaints or clinical errors or incidents. She does not want to mention alcohol in the letter (and does not want you to tell him about her querying his possible alcohol misuse) because it might "cause tensions at work", but she *does* want you to specifically rule out alcohol misuse.

iii. Sonia is an administrative assistant and David, her manager, has referred her to the OH department because she has been off work for the last month and has a fit note for a further month, stating "work-related stress". David mentions in the referral letter that she has never complained about stress at work and asks you what the real reason for her "alleged stress" is.

When Sonia attends her OH consultation, she tells you that she is suffering work stress as a result of bullying by her new manager, who had been appointed in his post six months previously. She felt that David continually belittled her in front of other colleagues and he "picked on her for anything", such as going to the toilet, which made her even more anxious about needing to go to the toilet. She had been worrying about coming into work and experiencing palpitations, nausea and dizziness. She had no other problems at work, and indeed had very much enjoyed her work since starting in that job three years ago. She now had problems sleeping, was overeating and had lost her confidence. The symptoms had steadily worsened over the last 3 months, and the turning point was when Sonia's mother discovered she had started to self-harm. Her mother insisted that Sonia go and see her GP, which she did. Sonia was now on anti-depressants and had started counselling, arranged by her GP. She had been reticent about coming to see you, but her GP encouraged her to do so. She is still worried about what you would say to David. She had also asked her GP not to mention "bullying" on her fit note, as she feared this could make things worse for her once she resumed work.

iv. Ernie is a supervisor in a chemical manufacturing factory. He was referred following a fall from a ladder, while he was working a night shift a week ago. He has sustained a shoulder soft tissue injury, for which he is having physiotherapy, paid for by his employer. His manager has referred him only for you to assess whether he is fit to resume work, and if so, in what capacity.

Ernie attends the consultation with his wife. They are concerned about his situation. He discloses to you that he went dizzy on the ladder, and this was probably the cause of his fall. He hopes you will not mention this to his manager, because he thinks the company might stop paying for physiotherapy if they knew that this was the cause of his fall. He is also worried he might lose his job if he is found unfit to work.

During his assessment, you note that he has poorly controlled type 2 diabetes and reports having experienced dizziness on exertion and on standing up quickly, for the last two years. On examination, he has a marked postural drop in his blood pressure, which you believe could well explain his dizzy spells. You feel that his symptoms could be improved with the correct treatment, so you advise him to see his GP, who you hope will refer him to a specialist. We will consider the ethical issues, including what you might write in your report, in the next sub-section. I also later use this case vignette as an example (in Chap. 9) to illustrate how I use an ethical reflection and audit tool (ERATOH: Ethics Reflection & Audit Tool in Occupational Health). This example can be found at Appendix 5 and I discuss the wider (that is, beyond just the immediate report) ethical issues of this case in Chap. 9 where I describe how this tool can be used.

Ethical Concerns Raised by the Case Vignettes

In each case, you will have explained your role as an OH practitioner, discussed the referral letter with the worker, and explained that you would be writing a report to the manager (and HR if this is the usual arrangement) to give your advice, at the end of the consultation. We will assume that in each case, the worker gave informed consent for the consultation to proceed, but we will look at different scenarios with regards to *permission to disclose* the report in each case. You will also have mentioned the limits of confidentiality, in particular, that you *have to* disclose relevant information if a third party might be at risk of harm if you did not disclose that information. Now let us turn to the specific ethical concerns that each vignette may help to illustrate.

i. Lorraine is already suffering from work-related ill-health, which may worsen if there was nothing done to alleviate her stressors. She does have responsibilities as a carer (for her mother), but she was offended that the head attributed her stress to that reason alone. Let us first think of the ethical implications of what we might do in practice, and then consider the ethical issues relevant to writing the report.

Our *primary* purpose as an OH professional is to protect her health. Workplace stressors pose a significant risk to her health and we are well placed to give advice that could reduce her stress. I suggest that our approach should be to advise at two levels: firstly, at organizational level, so that the employer can address the relevant psychosocial factors; and secondly, at a personal health level, to prevent Lorraine's condition deteriorating into a more severe stress illness.

The best approach to identifying and planning to manage work stressors is through a **risk assessment** approach. The school may already have a stress risk assessment tool. Otherwise you can point the head to relevant sources of information (for example, I have mentioned a UK resource in the Notes section). Typically, there are headings under which the significant stressors will be elicited, such as work demands, job role, control over work and so on. In Lorraine's case, work *demands* and recent *changes in her role* seem to be important sources of stress. In terms of stress management measures for role changes for example, the importance of appropriate *training* and adequate *support* to navigate these changes safely is usually highlighted. In addition to the obvious benefit that such a risk assessment approach usually gets to the *core* of the work-related stress (WRS) issues, it does so in an objective way, which makes it easier for all parties to engage in finding solutions in a more co-operative manner. In some countries and regions, carrying out risk assessments for Health and Safety risks (including psychosocial ones) is also a legal requirement.

Turning now to personal health advice, it is good that she has already engaged with her GP. From the description I have given above, she probably does not need medication at this stage. It is understandable that she might not feel counselling would be helpful, as to her (and probably you as well) the source of her stress seems obvious, and the priority should be to address the causes of the WRS. However, it may still be worth discussing with her whether seeing a counsellor during this difficult time could be helpful. She might benefit from support while she goes through the interviews and other interactions with the head (and possibly HR) to carry out the stress risk assessments and the follow-ups from these. This may be especially the case if you have access to a counselling service through the OH department, as such counsellors are usually more attuned to workplace issues. However, even if she sees a counsellor through her GP, she may also explore other coping strategies, including coping better with her home situation: For example, could others help with her mother's care? Would she benefit from some assertiveness techniques or training? However, it would probably be better for the counsellor to discuss these with her, as our most important contribution as OH professionals will be to help the organization address the WRS through a risk assessment approach. You may wish to mention other self-help techniques, including exercise, if her GP has not already done so.

If we now consider the report to be written to the manager, the main focus of your advice should be on helping her and the organization resolve the main source of concern to her (and threat to her health), which is her WRS. This is in line with our primary duty of protecting her health at work. Could this primary duty come into conflict with other ethical duties, such as confidentiality? In Lorraine's case as I have described it, I think probably not. It is likely that Lorraine will be thankful for the interest you have in her WRS and will understand your reasons for recommending that a stress risk assessment be undertaken. So, I believe that it is likely that she would give her permission for you to disclose your report. It is still important that she understands what your report will say. I would say to the headteacher that Lorraine suffers stress, and there is a significant contribution from work to her stress. If her WRS is not reduced, then there would be a risk of further deterioration in her health. My recommendation is that he (and HR if they are usually involved with this) carry out a WRS risk assessment to identify and manage the relevant stressors. I would, with Lorraine's agreement, mention that the areas of *work demands* and *changes in her role* merit particular attention (along with the consequent control measures which would usually include appropriate support and training). If Lorraine has agreed to attend counselling, I would also mention this so that the head can agree with her the times for her to attend her counselling appointments. I would not mention any details of her personal life, except to acknowledge that there are also some home stressors (especially as he already knows of her mother's dementia). By writing the report in this way, I would be honoring the relationship of trust (in this quasi-therapeutic relationship, which is fiduciary in nature—see Chap. 2) and disclosing only pertinent information. Remember (from Chap. 4) that confidentiality is concerned with *both* the relationship and the information disclosed in that relationship of trust.

In this scenario, it is unlikely that Lorraine would refuse PTD (permission to disclose) this report. If she did, I would try to understand her concerns and address these as best I could. I would point out that the situation at work would be unlikely to improve without some intervention such as a WRS risk assessment. Without a report, the head could take management action that was unhelpful to her. However, I would still respect her choice if she did not want this report released to the head and an HR professional.

A further scenario that is highly **unlikely** in Lorraine's case is her being a danger to students in her present state. However, one could envisage situations where a teacher had deteriorated to the extent that she started developing paranoid beliefs or thoughts of self-harming (maybe this ideation extending to students). In such situations, one **must** disclose a relevant report even without the teacher's PTD, because of the risk of harm to vulnerable parties. This eventuality would be covered in the early stages of a consultation, where we explain the limits of confidentiality, that is, when we would have to breach confidentiality if there were significant risk of harm to others. I mention this for completeness, as I do not believe that Lorraine would be in this situation at this stage.

ii. In Ashley's case, I would suggest that we should act **before** the consultation, by contacting his manager to explain our difficulties with her request *not* to inform Ashley of her concern about a possible alcohol issue. If we aim to be open, transparent and honest in our relationships with workers (and others), then I think the manager's not sharing her concerns about his misuse of alcohol is a major problem for us. How can we be open and honest with Ashley if we are keeping vital information from him? How can we obtain valid informed consent to the assessment when we are not divulging to him the true purpose of this consultation? I do not believe that this is possible, which is why I believe we should contact the manager to explain the difficulties in her proposed approach, and hopefully obtain her agreement that Ashley would be informed of the *real* reason for the referral. Ideally, this would be by the manager herself prior to the consultation, but if this is not possible, then you would share with Ashley what she has told the OH department, and she would then have a follow-up conversation with Ashley at the earliest opportunity afterwards.

There may some objections to my advice above, maybe based on patient safety arguments. However, I would counter this by pointing out that if there were sufficient management concerns over patient safety, the manager should act on these concerns and suspend him from clinical work pending investigation of the concerns (which would include an OH referral). At least this would be a more honest approach and the organization's alcohol policy, for example, could be applied.

I must also point out that there are practical problems, as well as the ethical ones, that arise if the "covert" approach to finding out if he had an alcohol problem. Most of the evidence of alcohol misuse comes from a truthful account of one's alcohol consumption. Only some of those who chronically abuse alcohol will show abnormal liver function tests, for example. Such testing in turn raises further ethical problems. How would you obtain valid consent for testing?

Although in this chapter we are mainly concerned with the report written following an assessment, I wanted to highlight with this case vignette the importance of framing the referral in an ethical way at the outset. In Ashley's case, once the reasons for the consultation are openly and honestly discussed with him, there is a greater likelihood of obtaining his informed consent for the assessment and permission to disclose the subsequent report. However, you should also stress that if there were patient safety concerns, you might have to disclose the report without his permission.

If the manager did not agree to you disclosing her concern about alcohol to Ashley, then I would be unhappy to proceed with a consultation at all. However, in agreement with your OH manager, you may decide to carry out a consultation but ignore the unwritten question about alcohol. As I have mentioned above, if the ward manager has sufficient concerns about the possibility of patient safety, then she would be responsible for investigating the concerns and even suspending Ashley from patient contact until investigations were completed.

Let us assume that the ward manager *does* understand the ethical position here and agrees for you to be open with Ashley about her concerns about his drinking. The content of your report would then depend on what Ashley admits to you. If he does admit to a problem with alcohol, then you are able to advise that the alcohol policy be applied. You would make a clinical assessment of any danger to patients and report on this. If he is temporarily not safe to work with patients, then there should be a plan of when he might be safe to do so and what he would need to do to achieve fitness to work with patients. This would include him giving a commitment to comply with necessary treatment, such as from his GP, specialist alcohol services or other specialist services.

If he does not admit to having an alcohol problem, then that is what you would report. Whether you suggest any blood testing would depend on your OH departmental practice. If he does smell of alcohol at work, then you could suggest to his manager that "for cause" alcohol testing, such as a breath test, could be used. This is usually done independently of OH, mainly because it would be difficult for OH professionals to have a supportive and rehabilitative role on the one hand, *and* simultaneously a policing and enforcing role on the other. However, I recognize that local arrangements do vary widely, so act in accordance to your local alcohol policy, to which the senior OH professionals should have had significant input.

Whether Ashley has an alcohol problem or not, you would be able to discuss this openly with him, if we assume that his manager has agreed to disclosing her concerns to him. Your report to the manager would then be able to reflect your findings and advice in an open and honest way, and Ashley would understand what you are advising and why (as opposed to the manager's initial approach, which was to try to find out about a possible alcohol problem *covertly*). An open and transparent approach engenders and maintains better trust by workers in OH services in the long run, which is essential if we are to protect their health. I would even suggest that such an open and honest approach is more likely to achieve *patient* (or other third party) safety, because if workers do not trust us, they are more likely to *conceal* their health issues, which could then deteriorate to the point that their patients would be at risk of harm.

iii. I have described Sonia's case to illustrate the problems we can face if we write a report to the manager who is in fact the alleged *perpetrator* of bullying. We face similar problems if the manager is alleged to be the perpetrator of any other form of discrimination or harassment. How you address such a problem may be constrained by your local arrangements, such as whether you can have access to anyone else in the organization, such as a senior manager or HR. This may be easier if you work as part of an in-house OH service, and more difficult if you work in an OH service that is outsourced, with little contact with the organization. However, even in the latter case, it may be possible to contact some relevant senior person (including HR) to whom you would address your report, instead of the alleged offender.

This is important, because otherwise Sonia may be fearful that David, her manager would use the information you provide *against* her, or simply ignore it and make life even more difficult for her. Some managers may not be aware of the impact of their behavior on others and be quite willing to change when they realize this. Others may not accept any criticism and become defensive, which then leads to increased tensions at work. We cannot always foresee the outcome of our advice, but at least if there is third party (hopefully objective) involvement, then there would be a better chance of an improvement in the work situation.

Sonia has already done as much as she can do to improve her health, in following the advice of her GP, taking medication and engaging with counselling. However, it is unlikely that her health would improve significantly unless the work situation were improved. In addition, although she might improve sufficiently to return to work with the help of her GP and counsellor, if she returned to work with the same bullying (whether real or perceived), it is very likely that her health would deteriorate again. Given that our primary purpose is to protect the health of workers, we should aim to give advice which can ameliorate the work situation. It is probable, I think, that Sonia would welcome your suggestion to contact someone other than David. While your report is being written and sent to the appropriate party, there may be other workplace avenues for her to explore, such as whether she would speak to her union representative and/or HR. Some organizations also operate a helpline (usually run by an external agency) in cases of bullying, which she may find helpful.

As to the content of you report, I think this should be brief. It would be addressed to the agreed third party (senior manager and/or HR) stating that Sonia reports bullying from her manager, David. I would mention that Sonia is doing everything she can to improve her health with the help of her GP, including medication and counselling, but that without some suitable intervention at work her health may not improve, and may in fact deteriorate if she faced the same work situation on resuming work. Appropriate interventions could include meetings with HR, followed by meetings between Sonia and David, possibly with mediation support if this available. The aim should be to have an agreed plan of how the working relationship between Sonia and David could be improved when she returns.

In terms of permission to disclose this report, I would expect Sonia to be happy to do this, as she would understand its purpose. However, if she did have any worries after the first consultation, this might be because she feels particularly vulnerable after her experiences at work.

I suggest that a follow-up meeting with yourself, maybe accompanied by a person she feels comfortable with for support, for example a relative or partner, or her trade union representative, will give her a better chance to assimilate what is being proposed, and decide whether to give her permission to disclose your intended report. The alternatives, which would be not to mention the workplace bullying, or not to send a report at all (stating that she had not given permission to disclose the report), are not likely to be in her interests. Such discussions between Sonia, her accompanying person and you are best when there is trust between all parties (see for example, "Relational Autonomy" in Chap. 3), which is why we should strive to improve worker trust in OH services.

iv. As I have mentioned above, I will later use Ernie's case to illustrate (in Chap. 9) how I use an ethical reflection tool (ERATOH) to identify and evaluate the ethical issues that arise, in a more comprehensive manner. Here I would like to concentrate mainly on the ethical issues that link with the OH report that we write to his manager after our assessment following the management referral.

On the face of it, this could be a simple assessment of Ernie's fitness to resume work, as this is the only question his manager has asked. Assuming that as a supervisor he has supervisory and administrative duties, then he could resume in that capacity as soon as he is sufficiently pain-free and not suffering side-effects from his analgesia (such as not experiencing drowsiness), probably within the next few days. However, he would be temporarily restricted from heavy manual duties until his shoulder had satisfactorily recovered. You could arrange a follow-up assessment, say in about four weeks, to review his shoulder symptoms and function, to advise whether he would then be fit to resume manual duties as well, or whether there need be a further temporary period of restriction. For example, he might no longer respond to physiotherapy or he might need further specialist treatment. From a practical perspective, as OH practitioners we are often drawn to the safety critical aspect of our consultations as a priority. This is entirely correct and laudable. In Ernie's case, whatever other advice we may give the manager, we would ensure that we mention that Ernie should not work at heights or in other work situations where his dizziness might endanger himself or others. However, this scenario does allow us to explore different layers of ethical concerns. We will do this both here and in Chap. 9: we will mainly focus on the ethical issues around *causation* here; we will look at the ethical implications of the *safety critical* aspects of his role and the practical management of this vignette (such as writing to his GP) further in Chap. 9.

One of the more difficult ethical questions in this case vignette is the concern that Ernie and his wife expressed at the start of the consultation: Should you mention in your letter that Ernie had experienced dizziness and that this could have led to his fall from the ladder? I do not believe that there is a right or wrong answer to this question. I will describe my stance on this but accept that others could take the opposite view. My view is that the manager has not asked about *causation*, so I would not mention this in my report. The only exception would be if I felt there were a significant risk of harm to others by my not mentioning this. I am balancing my fiduciary duty to Ernie against my duty to the employer, in deciding whether to give the additional information *at this stage*. I say "at this stage" because if Ernie's problems do not resolve, then there would be longer-term implications for his fitness for **all** his duties, so more information would likely need to be disclosed (see below). However, in this current report, I feel that disclosing the possible cause of Ernie's fall may cause him harm and would not greatly benefit the employer (namely, not paying for physiotherapy treatment). So, for me the balance points to *not* disclosing, although I can understand that others might prefer to disclose.

In taking this course of action, I would be open with Ernie about my reasons, and explain that if there had been a risk to others, then I would have needed to disclose this. In addition, if his condition did not improve after further treatment, he might then pose a health and safety risk to others (such as needing to be rescued if he fell in a vessel) if he resumed his full duties, and I would need to disclose the nature of his incapacities to his employer at that point.

In the current scenario, there is still a possibility that his symptoms could resolve after treatment from a specialist (assuming his GP does refer him to one). If this were the case, then Ernie would eventually be fit for all his duties, with no restrictions at work. I would mention this in my present report. However, there is still uncertainty about the longer term, so there would need to be further review appointments and further reports. Although in this first report I do not feel that I need to mention Ernie's dizziness symptoms, I would explain to him that if they persisted in the longer term, I would then need to explain the nature of his functional limitations (probably not working at heights or driving, for example). If, as a consequence, the employer asked me whether the symptoms could have contributed to his fall, I would have to tell the truth. My fiduciary duties to Ernie do not extend to *lying* to the employer. Furthermore, some might argue that not telling the employer all the facts initially still infringes the duty of veracity I owe to the employer (by omission). As I have previously explained, it is difficult to be certain of *which* of the moral principles or values we ought to give priority to in any given difficult situation in practice, and this is what I have aimed to show with this example. We need to weigh up the relevant moral principles in each situation and do the best we can in the circumstances. This includes reflecting on such cases and discussing these with colleagues (see Chap. 9).

I think it is important that we also protect Ernie's privacy by not writing unnecessary clinical and personal information. I would not normally mention Ernie's diabetes or drop in blood pressure unless there were a good reason to do so, and with Ernie's permission. The **functional** effects of any condition that can affect fitness for work, such as loss of awareness or consciousness **are** relevant to the employer, especially in safety critical work, and should be disclosed (this is discussed further in Chap. 9). It is by being open with and explaining to workers our rationale for what information we include in the report, that we can maintain their trust in us and OH services generally.

In writing MR reports, we should be conscious of our duty of confidentiality to the worker, but this must be balanced with the need to give the employer appropriate and relevant information. Sometimes these duties come into conflict. I have described my preferred course of action in Ernie's case but accept that this approach can be criticized. We should take any such criticism positively, reflect on why there can be divergent views in such cases and learn from the differences in opinion.

In this example, I have made the point that as the employer did not ask about causation, we did not have to address the issue of causation. However, I do not wish to give the impression here that we should *only* answer questions put to us in a management referral letter, despite my approach in Ernie's case. Indeed, there are occasions where an employer does specifically *not* ask advice about workplace adjustments or health and safety (H&S) risks, for example, but we feel that the advice is relevant for the manager to be able to address a workplace situation to protect a worker's health at work. I would go even further than this. I have encountered situations where the employer has said they did **not** wish to receive such advice! On those occasions, I feel we **should** give this advice even when it is not requested.

In the case of H&S advice, I think it will usually be straightforward enough to point to local H&S regulations and laws that would require us to discharge such professional duties (such as advising that risk assessments need to be reviewed and/or exposure assessments be carried out). I have found that it is with the second situation, that is, with regards workplace adjustments, that colleagues have more problems convincing the employer that they *should* be giving this advice (even if not requested by the manager). Typically, employers who do not want to receive advice on adjustments may say that these are too impractical/expensive/time consuming to implement. Another oft heard complaint from managers is that the worker, having had sight of the OH report, then expects the adjustments to be fully implemented. When this worker later finds that his manager tells him that it is not possible/too expensive/impractical to implement the adjustments as advised by OH, this then creates worker-employer conflict. The latter criticism is not unsurmountable: we ought to make it clear to the worker that our report to the manager is only **advisory** and it is up to the manager to decide what can be put in place in practice, subject to resource constraints and maybe the effect on other workers and so on.

Why do I think it is so important for us to give appropriate advice (either H&S or on adjustments) to employers? This is because the **primary aims** of OH are to protect workers' health and to help them remain at work where possible. We should make it clear to employers when they employ us or contract our services that this is a **fundamental** aspect of our duties. If we remained silent on these points when we could protect the health of workers (in the case of H&S advice) or help them remain at work with appropriate adjustments, then we would be behaving unethically.

To summarize the section on management referral (MR) reports, we can see how this very *practical* topic, an activity most of us do each working day, can bring to the fore many of the ethical issues we discussed in the theoretical chapters. In particular, this topic helps us look at theoretical concepts such as our dual obligations to workers and employers (Chap. 2), consent (both informed consent and permission to disclose), autonomy and trust (Chap. 3) and confidentiality and privacy (Chap. 4) in real life OH situations. To illustrate these, I have used four case vignettes to help us explore some of the more challenging areas of our practice such as work-related stress (WRS) and the use of risk assessments (Lorraine); information given by a manager "off the record" (Ashley); a referral by a manager who is the perpetrator of health harming behavior himself (Sonia); and whether we need to disclose information in our report that a manager did not ask about (Ernie).

I encourage you to consider my illustrations **critically**. My approaches to these challenges should be considered context-specific and not as necessarily "gold standard" responses to these. I hope that the fact that I have explained the underlying moral arguments for my preferred courses of action in each of these examples will help you when you are faced by similar but slightly different challenges. You will thus be better prepared to address the practical and moral issues you face in your OH practice that arise in writing MR reports, especially in the more difficult situations.

Ill-Health Retirement Reports

By ill-health retirement (IHR) reports, I mean those reports written for the purposes of advising a pension fund whether the applicant (current or ex-employee) meets the fund criteria of eligibility for early payment of their pension on the grounds of ill-health. The report is usually addressed to a pension fund manager but may also be to the employer who then forwards the report to the pension fund trustees. In some countries, this activity is carried out by insurance medicine physicians rather than OH physicians, but I think the same ethical principles would apply. Even in situations where OH physicians are conducting the IHR assessment and writing the report, it is best practice that this physician be **independent** of the worker or ex-employee (that is, the *applicant* to the pension fund) and the employer, if this is practically possible (see Chap. 2 regarding OH professional roles). This independence helps to remove real or perceived conflicts of interest when giving the advice on eligibility for IHR, especially as the outcome can entail the payment of significant amounts of money (cumulatively over the lifetime of the pension being paid). Although malingering and illness deception are probably **rare** in OH practice (see reference 6 in the Notes), these may occur more often in this area of practice than in other OH situations. It is more likely that applicants might exaggerate their symptoms, consciously or unconsciously, given the potential financial gains from being awarded an IHR. This is also be an area of OH practice where there might be more complaints from applicants, especially if their applications are unsuccessful.

I think it helps if we are completely transparent about our role when we are doing an IHR assessment and report, namely that this role requires **independence** from both the applicant and the employer (and communicate this to both parties very clearly). As we saw in Chap. 2, the OH professional in this role *cannot* have the same fiduciary obligations as in the therapeutic or quasi-therapeutic roles. Our primary duty here is to give objective and unbiased advice to the pension fund. We cannot properly perform this task if there is undue pressure or coercion from either the applicant or the employer.

In the independent OH role, we still have some of the fiduciary obligations: we should not profit from our position and we should have no conflicts of interest. We also have a duty of confidentiality, which we discharge by writing only relevant information in our report and disclose it to only the appropriate parties (usually to a pension fund manager, or to the employer who then transmits the report to the pension fund trustees), with a copy of the report to the applicant at the same time. I believe that in this role, we obtain both the applicant's informed consent to carry out the assessment **and** permission to disclose that report to the appropriate recipient at the *outset*, that is, at the start of the consultation. A system that would allow an IHR applicant to suppress an unfavorable report after the OH professional had reached her unbiased professional opinion is unethical in my view, as such a system could, for example, allow public funds to be misused. The IHR assessment process, including the fact that a report cannot be suppressed or altered (save for factual corrections), must be clearly explained to the applicant *before* the assessment. Such problems could be mitigated if employers strictly adhered to pension fund rules and regulations, which might (and in my opinion, **should**) highlight the need for the OH professional to be independent. If an employer had not correctly followed the pension scheme processes, then the OH professional should decline conducting the assessment and offering an opinion.

Self-referral Reports

By self-referral report, I mean a report that might arise following a self-referral by a worker to an OH professional. The ability to self-refer to OH services varies from organization to organization. In the UK it seems to me that the ability for a worker to self-refer is becoming less available and workers are usually advised to approach their manager or HR to be referred to the OH service. In some cases, this might deter them from seeking an appointment with the OH professional at all, especially if it is a sensitive matter that they wish to discuss. I understand that there are OH resource and operational constraints, so it may be difficult to accommodate too many OH appointments. However, I believe that the ability for workers to self-refer can engender greater trust in an OH service, as we might be perceived as being more "neutral", that is, available for advice to both the employer **and** workers (see Chap. 2 for comments on worker trust in OH). I would further argue that giving workers reduced (or more difficult) access to OH could diminish our ability to fulfill one of our core aims, which is to protect the health of workers at work.

When we do see a worker who has self-referred, in my view, this will usually be in a *quasi-therapeutic* type of relationship (see Chap. 2). This is at the other end of the spectrum of OH professional-worker relationships compared to the *independent* one described above (in IHR assessments). I have previously explained (in Chap. 2) that this type of interaction with a worker is the closest one to a therapeutic relationship, so we **do** owe the worker all the fiduciary obligations in this role.

Although we are looking at report writing in this chapter, not all self-referral consultations will entail a report being written. This would be a matter of choice for the worker. The only exception would be if other parties could be harmed or be put at risk by non-disclosure, which should be made clear to the worker who self-refers at the beginning of the consultation. However, there are many instances where it would be in the worker's interest for a report to be written to a relevant party, such as his manager or HR. For example, if the worker's health were suffering or at risk by some aspect of his work, then a report highlighting the workplace problem(s) is often the best way to have an amelioration of the situation. I would point this out to the worker, but the final decision is his. Sometimes, he needs some time to reflect on the proposed course of action or the report, and I would encourage him to take this time. On other occasions, he might benefit from some counselling sessions (for example in cases of workplace bullying) before he is ready to engage in a process with his manager or HR to address the issues at work. Once again, I would delay writing and sending a report until he is ready. The content of the report and who it is sent to would also be matters to agree with him. Sometimes it would be inappropriate to write to his immediate manager (such as in cases where the latter were the source of reported bullying, see Sonia's example earlier in this chapter), and in such cases a report might be sent to a more senior manager or to HR. The report content, as usual, should be concise and as objective, factual and unbiased as possible. This is because we should act in such a fashion that OH is trusted by both, the workers and the employer.

Case Conferences

Another instance where communication in OH practice can lead to ethical difficulties is when this is carried out *verbally*. This communication could be, for example, in the form of a phone call from a manager or HR to clarify what an OH professional wrote in her report about a worker's fitness for work or sickness absence. As some authors have noted, this could lead to breaches of confidentiality and OH professionals must be careful about this. However, if the clarification is purely on information already contained in the report, then there would be no breach of confidence. I would make contemporaneous notes of that phone call or conversation to document what information had been exchanged. If the manager or HR put forward questions that I feel go *beyond* simple clarification of my advice (previously given), then I would ask that they request this further advice in writing, with a copy to the worker. If I feel my reply might disclose some new information, then I would also request the worker's permission to disclose the further advice, letting him see my proposed reply. It is important for all our communications to be transparent if we are to maintain the trust of the workforce in OH.

Sometimes the form of oral exchange is more elaborate and complex. For example, there can be meetings between a manager, HR and OH professionals to discuss a worker's sickness absence. Such meetings are often called "case conferences". I am aware that some OH colleagues are very wary of such meetings. They feel these are a potential ethical minefield where they might unwittingly breach confidence. However, case conferences are used extensively in some organizations, so we should be aware of how to participate in these in an ethical manner.

For case conferences to be carried out in an ethical way, they must be as transparent and open as possible, and maintain worker confidentiality, to ensure that OH services be worthy of worker (and employer) trust. So, it is essential that the worker is aware that a case conference to discuss his situation is being conducted. I would prefer it for the worker (and his representative if he wished) to be present at that meeting. I realize that this is not the practice in some organizations. In fact, on some of the occasions where the worker *has* been present, I have been dismayed at how intrusive the HR questions (addressed directly to the worker) were, and the worker himself divulged very personal and sensitive details beyond what any OH professional would likely have disclosed. On such occasions, I have had to point out that some of the questions were not appropriate. Therefore, although my preference is for the worker to be present, in practice this can be unnecessarily intrusive and distressing for the worker. I also have had positive experiences where I found managers and HR to be extremely understanding and the case conferences have resulted in beneficial outcomes for both the worker and the organization.

Some argue that for such consultations (case conferences) to be ethical, the consent of the worker should be obtained beforehand. I agree with this in principle. However, I find it difficult to see how this would be applied consistently in practice. What are we asking the worker to consent to? If it is simply to clarify information that the manager has received in a previous report, then I would argue that consent (or permission to disclose) is *not* required. However, if there is the possibility of **new** information being disclosed, could prior permission adequately cover this? Presumably the OH professional herself would not know what the information might be. I believe that this is the situation where it would be best to have the worker (and representative) present. In any case, it is essential to make the worker aware that this case conference will be taking place and to find a workable solution. If the worker cannot be present, then I would make sure that the manager and HR know that **only** information that they hold will be clarified with no new information being disclosed and explain this to the worker. I would make notes during the meeting. A summary agreed by all parties, should be made available to those present and the worker, after the meeting.

Conclusion

Communication is an important topic in OH practice. In this chapter we have looked at a range of written, as well as some oral, communications relevant to our practice. This has given us the opportunity to apply some of the theoretical concepts that we previously discussed, such as confidentiality, informed consent and permission to disclose information, in a variety of OH situations. The topics of IHR and self-referral reports also demonstrate the different ethical obligations that our OH roles, from the "quasi-therapeutic" to "independent" spectrum, can give rise to. I hope that my analyses of the more difficult (and sometimes contentious) examples will be of help to you in your ethical deliberations, when you confront similar situations.

Chapter 7
Health Surveillance

Introduction

Our primary aim is to protect and promote the health of workers at work, and "to sustain and improve their working capacity and ability". One activity that we carry out regularly and that fits well with this primary aim is *health surveillance*. I will use the term health surveillance to describe the activities we carry out to detect any ill-effects of *work on health*, as opposed to *health screening*, which does not necessarily imply an adverse work effect or harmful exposure. I will come back to this later. In addition, health surveillance is much more than just doing an assessment to detect changes in health status of individual workers. The information we gather and feed back to the employer (usually in the form of "grouped data") can help with their efforts to establish and maintain a safe and healthy working environment for the *collective* of workers, that is, health surveillance *should* be a vital element of the employer's **risk assessment** and risk management processes. However, for health surveillance to achieve these important aims, health surveillance programs need to be designed and conducted to good OH and evidence-based standards. I believe that poorly designed and poorly conducted health surveillance is intrinsically **unethical**, as I will explain later. Even health surveillance that is appropriately devised and carried out does raise ethical issues, even conflicts, at times. We will explore these ethical issues in greater depth as they arise *before*, *during* and *after* the health surveillance assessment is conducted.

Before the Assessment

As practitioners, we may be forgiven for maybe concentrating more on the ethical issues that could arise from the assessment itself. However, for our health surveillance activity to be ethical, we need to give significant and careful thought about *how* and *why* we should be doing such health surveillance, even before the worker presents

© Springer Nature Switzerland AG 2020
J. Tamin, *Occupational Health Ethics*,
https://doi.org/10.1007/978-3-030-47283-2_7

himself at our clinics for an assessment. I will group the ethical issues that we need to consider in this *pre*-assessment phase under the sub-headings of "planning a health surveillance program" and "information to workers" about the program.

Planning a Health Surveillance Program

The person planning and designing the health surveillance program must (i) be **competent** to do so; and (ii) have all the required information available to her. I think that she should be an OH professional with the required training, qualifications and expertise. I would not expect someone who did not that range and depth of knowledge to be able to plan such a program to the required standard. Given the possible invasive nature of the questions and investigations, the harms to workers that can result from over- or under-diagnosing occupational ill-health conditions, then it follows that it would be **unethical** to conduct a program that was not properly planned and overseen by a competent professional. Secondly, she needs access to **all** relevant information such as risk assessments (which should include information about all the workplace health hazards), which workers are exposed and the exposure patterns, results of exposure assessments (such as personal and environmental monitoring) and results of previous health surveillance if this has been carried out. In certain jurisdictions, the employer must also be made aware that if there were a "case" of occupational disease detected by such health surveillance, they would need to report this to the competent authority. For example, in the UK, they would need to report to the Health and Safety Executive (HSE) under the Reporting of Injuries, Disease and Dangerous Occurrences Regulations (RIDDOR). This could lead to an inspection and even prosecution by the HSE.

The ICOH Code stresses the importance of OH professionals being familiar with the work and working environment, and I agree that this is vitally important. Without an accurate appreciation of the actual working conditions, environment and practices, it would be possible for the OH professional in charge of designing the health surveillance program to misinterpret the workforce exposure to hazards, and therefore the program would be defective for that reason. I accept that a senior OH professional (who is likely to be in charge of the program) may not have the time to visit every workplace or work area. Instead, it may be necessary for a more junior OH professional to carry out some of the workplace visits, and report back to the senior colleague. This is also a crucial aspect of OH training, and we develop our skills in interpreting workplace hazards and so on by this carrying out this activity. For example, my OH colleagues will probably readily recall some workplace visits where they spotted a container of a chemical hazard not listed in the information provided by the organization! In my experience, such oversight by the employer is usually completely unintentional, but it takes a trained eye to spot such critical details. If workers are exposed to substances hazardous to health which have been missed from the information provided, then it follows that the health surveillance activity will not adequately contribute to their health protection. From a purely legal stand-point, it is possible for OH professionals to add a disclaimer to the effect that the health surveillance program is based on the information provided by the employer. But does this discharge our *moral* duty to protect the health of workers? I do not believe so. So, this is one reason that a workplace visit, as part of devising the health surveillance program, should be done by a trained OH professional who is able to correctly identify possible hazardous workplace exposures. Another situation where such a visit can be invaluable is when an OH professional can identify a group of workers who might not be thought to be exposed to a workplace hazard, but in fact *are* exposed. An example of this was the administrative staff of a manufacturing company. Based on their job titles and the information provided by the company, they were not initially thought to be at risk of exposure and were not included in the initial health surveillance plan. However, when an OH professional visited the work site, she immediately identified that the administrative staff were working in an area adjacent to the main manufacturing plant, and their office was in fact used as thoroughfare for managers and production workers to access other parts of the site! They were then included in the program, which included respiratory surveillance and biological monitoring. The biological monitoring results in fact did confirm a level of exposure in this group. It is true that if the company had employed professionals with occupational hygiene or health and safety expertise, they would likely have identified that this office should also (that is, in addition to the manufacturing areas) be subject to air and personal monitoring, and so on. But many smaller companies do not have this expertise in-house (and may not think of buying in such services). On a happier note, this company did relocate their administrative staff away from the main plant after receiving the OH advice that accompanied the health surveillance feedback.

Once the OH professional has all the required information, including from the workplace visit, she can then plan the health surveillance program. The first question she needs to ask herself is whether health surveillance *should* in fact be undertaken, that is, (i) whether there is worker exposure to hazards and (ii) whether there are valid techniques to detect any health effects.

(i) It may seem self-evident that health surveillance is only justified if there is like-lihood of worker exposure to workplace hazards. Indeed, it would be unethical to conduct such activity without good justification, given the intrusive nature of the questions and the possible negative outcomes of testing (we will return to this point later in the next section "The assessment"). Nonetheless, sometimes there may be commercial pressures to deliver "health surveillance" when there is no need for it (for example, to undertake audiometry in a work population *not* exposed to noise or Hand-Arm Vibration Syndrome [HAVS] screening when the employer has not conducted the necessary exposure and risk assessments!) and there is no regulatory requirement for such surveillance. As OH profession-als, we **must** strongly resist such pressures as it is clearly unethical (because we must uphold professional integrity) for us to carry out unwarranted health surveillance.

(ii) If it is established that there *is* significant worker exposure to hazard(s), the OH professional in charge of the health surveillance program must then determine whether there is a **valid** technique for assessing the health effect. To guide her in this deliberation, the well-known *Wilson and Jungner* criteria for health screening, either in its original version or the updated one in a WHO Bulletin, will be a very helpful checklist. However, we do need to modify these useful concepts to fit with our context of health surveillance, as we are screening for health effects related to specific work exposures. Sometimes, the requirement for health surveillance (assuming there is relevant exposure) may be specified by national or regional laws or regulations, so the issue of cost of screening versus cost of treatment for the condition, for example, is not one that usually concerns us. In terms of acceptability of the test to the population, if there is a choice of techniques, then the least invasive one should be chosen (for example, breath testing in preference to a blood test).

Information to Workers

It is important that management and workers are clear about the purpose of the health surveillance to be undertaken, what this will involve and how any affected worker will be handled by the employer. Ideally, worker representatives would be involved in these discussions with the employer, so that they and their members understand how and what results will be communicated (to workers and managers), what the consequences of refusing to have health surveillance could be, and what arrangements will be in place for any worker found to be affected, such as redeployment or relocation (away from the relevant exposure), whether temporary or permanent. It is important for workers themselves to understand the arrangements and agreements with their employer, as they are more likely to engage positively with the program when this is the case. But it is also important for the *OH professionals* to be aware of these agreements, so that they can give appropriate and correct information to individual workers prior to their assessment, for the informed consent to be valid.

Let us remind ourselves of the case of Billy (Chap. 3, "Informed consent") to illustrate what I mean by this. If you recall, the OH adviser, Kathryn, will be take a blood sample for serum lead as part of his surveillance. She needs to know, for example that if he had a high blood test result he would be suspended from lead work temporarily, probably by being relocated to an area of the factory where there is little or no exposure to lead. But another consequence (if this agreed by the managers and worker representatives) of a high blood lead could be a temporary restriction from working overtime. Billy may worry more about the financial consequences from this restriction and he needs to be made aware of this by Kathryn for his consent to be truly *informed*.

A final word before we move to the actual assessment itself: It is **essential** that all equipment used for the health surveillance program is properly calibrated and maintained, as basing advice and decisions on unreliable results **cannot** be ethical. If the OH service is active in the realm of quality systems and audit (which is to be encouraged), then there are usually systems in place to ensure the equipment used will be satisfactory and reliable.

The Assessment

The assessment must be carried out by a **competent** OH professional, that is, one with the required training and qualifications. It follows that this OH professional will be familiar with the workplace, the risks to health from this particular exposure, giving advice on safe working practices, as well as having been trained in the ethical requirements of obtaining consent, maintaining confidentiality and our primary duty of protecting the health of the worker. There are some countries and jurisdictions where there the OH professional must be specifically accredited or registered to undertake some forms of health surveillance, for example, for workers exposed to lead, asbestos or ionizing radiation. However, whether there is regulation and regulatory authority oversight or not, we have a **moral** obligation as OH professionals to ensure that we have the required competencies to carry out this important activity. Otherwise, the health of workers could be put at risk, maybe through under- or over-diagnosis of work-related ill-health, or false reassurance, or incorrect advice. One such example that comes to my mind is the case of a company doctor (without OH training) who, through his ignorance, arranged for workers exposed to *lead* to have annual chest x-rays for many years and never arranged blood lead testing! This was eventually picked up by a factory inspector. This may have been over 30 years ago, but it remains a salutary reminder that we cannot over-emphasize the importance of having *competent* OH professionals doing health surveillance.

Apart from the competence of the OH professional, the other major ethical issue we should consider during the assessment itself (or at least, at the start of the assessment) is that of the worker's **consent**. As I explained in Chap. 3, I view "consent" in our OH context as *two* consenting processes, namely *informed consent* (IC) and *permission to disclose* (PTD). This is because we first need the worker's IC to proceed with the assessment, and secondly the worker's PTD to disclose some information (which may be in the form of a fitness statement) to the employer. We will return to PTD in the next section. Here, I want to focus on the IC process, as this is what is relevant for us to be able to carry out this assessment. Of course, as part of the information given to the worker for the consent to be *informed*, we must mention that there would be information, based on the result of this assessment, given *to* the employer (in whichever form is applicable to this health surveillance context, as I will describe in the next section). However, if we recall (see Chap. 3), the main ethical justification for IC now centers on respect for the worker's **autonomy**. Other reasons for requiring IC are *voluntariness* (or freedom from coercion) and protecting *bodily integrity*. Of course, this concept of consent was originally articulated in the context of research on human participants, and then applied to the health care setting.

Therefore, we may wish to determine to what extent the same justifications would apply in our context of OH health surveillance.

There is very little in the way of health surveillance techniques that would make us too concerned about bodily integrity. Indeed, the most invasive procedure that we do is probably a venepuncture. However, to some workers, this may still be anxiety provoking, especially for those with a needle phobia. Moreover, if we extend the concept of bodily integrity to encompass a sense of *self*, including our genetic make-up, then genetic testing could be deemed to be protected by our concern for bodily integrity. Although genetic testing is not normally undertaken in OH practice, we must remain wary of pressures from employers and insurers to do this in future. We could also appeal to the more recognized concept of respect for the worker's autonomy, rather than protecting bodily integrity, to protect him from such unwarranted testing.

Returning to our health surveillance procedures, here our concern would be that the worker is attending the assessment *voluntarily* and *free from coercion*. Indeed, the ICOH Code reminds us of this. The ICOH Code uses the phrase: "non-coerced informed consent of the workers." Presumably, if we think there might be coercion, then we expect this would be from the employer. I have previously mentioned that if there is coercion, then consent **cannot** be valid (for example in Chap. 6). However, the reality may be more nuanced than this.

The employer has a duty to protect their workforce from the harmful effects of workplace exposures. Therefore, it could be argued that the employer has a legitimate right to insist that workers undergo health surveillance. In addition, for some jurisdictions there will be legal requirements to have health surveillance programs for some specific workplace hazards, such as ionizing radiation, asbestos, or lead. We must balance this interest in protecting the workforce with an individual worker's right to accept or refuse participation in the health surveillance program. In this context, our concerns about the workers not being coerced and our need to respect their autonomy are quite closely aligned. Indeed, freedom from coercion and respect for autonomy are the important reasons why we must obtain truly informed consent. However, what do we mean by coercion here?

We will have a further discussion about coercion in the next chapter (Chap. 8) when we consider the vaccination of workers. In the context of health surveillance, coercion seems to imply that the employer would force workers to undergo health surveillance against their wishes. This would be by means of threats of adverse consequences (such as dismissal) if they did not agree to be assessed for this purpose. Now, as OH professionals, this would be very disturbing circumstances under which we would be carrying out an assessment! We simply could not accept the worker's consent as being valid, so we would not be able to progress with the assessment itself. That is why it is so important to get the *pre*-assessment phase right. As mentioned previously, the program must be properly evidence-based and planned. But it is just as important that the whole process is transparent, and ideally have had worker or worker representative involvement in its formulation. This *participative* approach makes it much less likely that the employer might feel compelled to using a *coercive* one. It is therefore important that we, OH professionals, influence the employer and workers as much as we can to collaborate in designing a health surveillance program that both can trust and where the workforce willingly participates.

I think we also resist any coercive approaches because of our *respect for the worker's autonomy*, which is nowadays the most recognized justification for requiring the worker's informed consent (IC). I would now like to turn our attention to the *informed* part of IC. We touched on part of this in the pre-assessment sub-section, when we considered the importance of our being as fully aware as we can of the possible consequences of testing, so that we are able to convey this information to the worker. The example I used there (in the pre-assessment sub-section) was the possibility of Billy being restricted from working overtime if his blood lead result was high. More generally, the ICOH Code reminds us that "The potentially positive and negative consequences of participation in screening and health surveillance programmes should be discussed as part of the consent process." The positive consequences will include detecting any adverse health effect caused by work. Hopefully, this will be at an early stage and potentially reversible or curable. Workplace interventions such as removal from exposure to the health hazard, or other risk reduction measures (such as limiting the exposure, for example in the case of vibration, or enhanced protective measures, such as better level respiratory protection against dusts and fumes) will likely be part of the interventions aimed to improve or protect this worker's health. However, the measures designed to protect his health may also have negative consequences, such as financial ones, if redeployment to a safer job or work area is not possible. Hopefully there will be some insurance arrangements to mitigate against the financial hardships, but this is not always the case. There are also other possible negative consequences, such as false reassurance from false negatives, or unnecessary anxieties from false positives, but as these apply to all types of health screening, I will not address such consequences in detail here. What is important is for the OH professional to be knowledgeable on such matters, and to be open and honest in communicating to the worker the relevant consequences of having this assessment. At that point, with the worker's fully informed consent, it is ethically safe to proceed with the assessment itself.

After the Assessment

The most obvious ethical issues in the post-assessment phase center around *information exchanges*, that is, the OH professional providing the results of the assessment or advice based on these results to the worker and the employer. Sometimes, information must also be sent to third parties as well, such as regulatory bodies (depending on local laws and regulations), as previously mentioned. The key to addressing the ethical issues around this information exchange is to obtain the worker's *permission to disclose* (PTD) the result or advice. However, there are also some less obvious but important ethical issues at this stage of the process. I will discuss these below under the sub-heading of "quality issues". If our justification for subjecting workers to intrusive questioning and tests is that we are protecting their health, then is the assessment achieving this protection for the individual worker and the group of workers? If we fall short of achieving this desired health protection through our health surveillance process, then there is a strong argument that it would be unethical to conduct this health surveillance program at all.

Quality Issues

Health surveillance is an important OH activity, as it directly relates to protecting and maintaining the health of workers at work. However, for the program to be effective, we should ensure that we address certain issues (which I will call "quality issues") in this post-assessment phase. Indeed, if we do not, and the program is less than effective, in my opinion we would be acting unethically. I will describe the quality issues in turn:

(i) For the individual worker undergoing health surveillance, the data from the assessment should be used optimally. This means that any abnormal results should be reviewed by an OH professional with the required competence and expertise. This OH professional should also have access to all relevant data to make the best interpretation of this abnormal result. This includes relevant exposure data, such as environmental and personal monitoring results where available, as well as that particular worker's **previous** health surveillance results. Without such data, it is more difficult to evaluate the abnormal result and reach a diagnosis (for example, whether the health condition is likely to be work-related or not). The added value of previous health data of the individual worker is that sometimes there is a steady decrement over time that would otherwise go unnoticed, as they may well still fall within a population "normal". An example would be a small but steady reduction in lung function results over several years, which may indicate that the worker is developing chronic obstructive pulmonary disease from dust exposure at work, and this would not be otherwise identified without the availability of longitudinal data. I realize that if OH health surveillance is outsourced, different OH providers may hold data for different periods and may not want to share this. I would urge OH providers to work together to make such data available to one another, as it is in the interest of the workers they are looking after at different times. Another practice I would guard against is simply sending a worker with an abnormal health surveillance result to his GP (general practitioner, or family doctor), *without* any OH specialist evaluation. A GP does not usually have the OH expertise and training to correctly interpret this result, and in addition would not have the workplace data required to do so. It may be appropriate to send a worker to see his GP *after* the OH specialist has diagnosed the work-related condition, maybe for further evaluation and treatment from a medical specialist (at least, this is can be the case in the UK). We must be careful of practices that would not optimize the results of a health surveillance program for the individual worker. This ought to be planned prior to the assessment by the competent OH professional (as I have previously mentioned), but I have witnessed programs where this has not happened. The ethical justification for carrying out health surveillance is that this will contribute to protecting the health of the worker. If the intended protection does not occur through such system (or design) failures as I have just outlined, then that program is intrinsically unethical.

(ii) I now turn to the **collective** health of the group of workers undergoing health surveillance. The most effective way to protect their health from workplace hazards will probably be through the employer controlling and managing these hazards appropriately. Health surveillance information, for example in the form of aggregated health data from the assessments, can give valuable information as to whether the employer's risk assessments and control measures are functioning properly. Of course, it is important to keep the privacy of individual information by anonymizing this information. However, a **report** summarizing the relevant health surveillance findings (maybe by department or work area, but individual workers should not be identifiable) available to both the employer and workers will be an important contribution to safeguarding their health. It should be an intrinsic part of a health surveillance program.

(iii) There should be on-going regular reviews of health surveillance program itself to ensure it remains appropriate for the workforce, the work context and the hazards, as well as the techniques and methods used remain up-to-date and evidence-based. There should also be regular audits of different parts of the health surveillance process, for example, whether confidentiality is adequately protected, whether equipment is properly calibrated and maintained, and so on. Such quality improvement practices are essential ensure that a health surveillance program delivers what is intended, that is, to contribute to protecting the health of workers at work.

Conclusion

Health surveillance is a key OH activity. It is a way for us as OH professionals to help protect the health of workers. However, to achieve this vitally important objective, health surveillance must be properly designed and carried out by appropriately trained competent OH professionals. Health surveillance also raises some important ethical issues which we have discussed in this chapter. For example, it highlights the difficulties we can face from our duties to protect the health of workers (the principle of beneficence), as well as respecting their autonomy and their right to privacy. Sometimes these duties can be in conflict. However, these tensions can be alleviated if the program is designed and conducted with an open and participative (that is, worker participation) approach. It is also crucially important that we ensure that the opportunities for worker health protection are optimized, both at the individual and collective levels. If we do so, we will be carrying one of our core activities effectively and ethically.

Chapter 8
Vaccinations

Introduction

This is the third (and final) chapter where we will be drawing on the insights gained from our ethics theory chapters to help us better understand the ethical issues arising from our OH practice. Vaccinations are an important OH activity, that many practitioners will be involved with (some more than others). Vaccinations also raise some ethical problems that can be analyzed from a somewhat different perspective, compared with those we have encountered so far in the practical section. There will be different ethical issues that arise, depending on the context and the reasons for a vaccination program. The most striking difference in terms of ethical analysis arises when an individual is vaccinated for the benefit of *others*. However, vaccinations given for population health reasons (that is, again for the benefit of others) are commonplace in the discipline of Public Health (PH). So, those vaccinations (in PH) may raise problems similar to those we encounter in OH. In PH, these ethical questions are addressed in a branch of ethics known as "Public Health ethics". We will first see how these issues are considered in PH ethics, and then see whether the analyses in PH ethics can help with our understanding of the ethical problems that we might encounter with OH vaccinations.

Vaccinations and Public Health Ethics

Vaccination programs at population level can have different primary aims, such as:

(i)   to protect the individual, e.g. tetanus;
(ii) to protect specific at-risk groups, e.g. influenza ("flu") vaccine for diabetics, those with respiratory diseases and the elderly;
(iii) to protect a community by achieving "population immunity" (also known as "herd immunity"), e.g. measles and rubella.

© Springer Nature Switzerland AG 2020
J. Tamin, *Occupational Health Ethics*,
https://doi.org/10.1007/978-3-030-47283-2_8

(iv) In addition, there are occasional vaccination programs to deal with a specific outbreak, e.g. a flu pandemic.

The type of program that raises the most ethical issues and is debated the most in PH ethics literature is usually the one listed at (iii) above, that is, the one that aims to achieve **herd immunity**. In this type of program, there may or may not be some benefit to the individual being vaccinated, but the main aim is to achieve a certain proportion of vaccinated individuals in a population, for the benefit of that *population as a whole*. Let us consider the following two examples to explain this further, and especially to describe the possible ethical tensions and even conflicts that can arise. In the first example, vaccination confers benefit to the individual who is vaccinated, whereas in the second there is negligible or no benefit for the vaccinated individual:

(a) We will first look at measles vaccination. Measles infection is usually a short-lived acute illness, but on occasion there can be serious complications, such as pneumonia, meningitis and encephalitis. There are some vulnerable groups, such as young children, the elderly and immunocompromised patients, who are at higher risk of developing such complications. Now, the measles vaccine is often administered as part of a combined "measles, mumps and rubella" (MMR) vaccine, so my ethical analysis of measles vaccination may appear not to be reflecting actual practice. However, I would argue that it is irrelevant that three vaccines are given together: there can still be an ethical discussion for each of the *individual* vaccines, and each of these discussions may be different, as we will see in the examples that I have chosen (my second example being rubella, see below). For measles vaccination, there is an individual *as well as* a population benefit. This is because the vaccine protects the vaccinated individual from an infection with possible serious complications and each individual who is vaccinated increases the vaccinated proportion within a community, which will help to achieve herd immunity.

(b) The second example is the rubella vaccine. As we noted above, it is usually given as part of MMR vaccination. Rubella infection itself is a mild disease, but the concern is the severity of the effects it can have on a **fetus** if the mother contracted the infection. The reason for aiming for a high uptake of rubella vaccination is to protect the fetus through herd immunity (through maternal immunity). In the UK, rubella vaccination was given to girls and women only, but this strategy was not successful as pregnant women still became infected with rubella. So, the rubella vaccination program was extended to include males to achieve herd immunity, although there is **no** benefit for the vaccinated males themselves.

We will now consider some of the ethical points which the two examples set out above raise:

(i) If we look at vaccination from an individual perspective, then it could be understandable why men and boys might decline being vaccinated against rubella. This is a rather short-sighted view, as their participation in the program could benefit of their own children (or future children) at some point. Even if they do not have children, it would benefit the communities in which they live. There-fore, although a narrow interpretation of autonomy might justify a decision to refuse vaccination, a more reflective and relational articulation of autonomy would not (see Chap. 3, "Relational autonomy"). Moreover, if we take the value of solidarity into account, then we would hope that males would feel equally engaged in protecting the future children of that community.

(ii) The second ethical issue that such examples raise is known as the "free-rider" issue. Let us take the measles example to explain this. If Malcolm refuses to be vaccinated against measles, and his community happens to have attained herd immunity anyway, Malcolm is then protected because of the herd immunity. This holds true unless Malcolm travels to another area where there is no such herd immunity, or if someone with the live virus from outside that community came into contact with Malcolm. But otherwise, Malcolm would benefit from the herd immunity to measles of his community, but not has not accepted any of the risks and discomforts (albeit minor) of having the vaccine. This is why he would be deemed to be a "free-rider" in that situation. The Nuffield Council on Bioethics consider such a view to be unhelpful, as the situation with vaccines is generally more complex. Malcolm may have other concerns about the vaccine and may not even realize he would benefit from herd immunity. I agree with the Nuffield Council that the "free-rider" issue is not one which should concern us much, but I mention it because it is often a point that is raised in this context.

(iii) A third and more significant ethical issue is whether those who refuse vaccina-tion could be *coerced* into accepting it, and whether that coercion be morally defensible. This is an issue that is also relevant to us in OH practice, as we will see later (in the next section). Now, I have previously explained (for example in Chap. 3) that coercion is generally unacceptable, which is why we put so much emphasis on obtaining **consent**, fully informed and voluntarily given. However, could a public interest in protecting the community override this? The Nuffield Council on Bioethics opined that there are two situations where "quasi-mandatory" measures could be justified: for serious contagious dis-ease (such as smallpox) and for eradication of serious disease if "eradication is within reach". What is meant by "quasi-mandatory measures" is that the individual refusing the vaccine would suffer some detriment. For example, in some countries, if children are not vaccinated against certain diseases, then they cannot attend schools. The discussion is generally very nuanced and takes careful account of the harms and benefits of each action. Commentators make it clear that voluntariness is the preferred approach in vaccination programs, but there is also good consensus that where a voluntary approach does not provide sufficient numbers of vaccinated individuals to achieve herd immunity, then some form of coercion could be considered, for the benefit of the community. This is an important point to take into our consideration of vaccinations in OH practice.

Vaccinations and OH

There are some similarities with the ethical issues between vaccinations done in the OH setting, compared with PH vaccinations. However, there are also some differences. In this section, we will explore these ethical issues, with particular emphasis on the differences with PH ethics.

Before we do so, it is worth reflecting on how performing vaccinations may differ from the rest of our OH practice. In many countries, OH has a primarily preventive role, and in those countries, the activity closest to a therapeutic activity might arguably be performing a vaccination. For most of our activities, we are giving advice in some form, and *permission to disclose* relevant information is the predominant ethical issue. With vaccinations, it is the other consenting process, namely *informed consent*, that is at the forefront of our ethical considerations. Vaccinations also differ from another interventional OH activity such as venipuncture, in that we introduce a substance in the worker's bodily systems. This substance could have some potential for some harm. Therefore, accurate and relevant information about the possible harms (as well as the benefits) of that substance need to be explained to the worker for his consent to be properly informed.

Now, returning to the types of vaccinations in OH, there are some similarities and some differences with those given for PH reasons. They can be grouped as follows:

(i)   For the protection of the individual worker, such as with travel vaccines which many OH departments administer.
(ii)   For the protection of the worker *and* of others. This includes hepatitis B and varicella (chickenpox) vaccinations in healthcare workers (HCWs), for their own protection and patient protection.
(iii) Primarily for the protection of specific at-risk groups. This includes vaccinating HCWs against rubella to protect the fetus of a pregnant patient, and against influenza ('flu') to protect elderly patients.

The ethical issues arise primarily in situations (ii) and (iii), which we will discuss further. As these ethical issues are slightly different in each of the examples, we will consider each one in turn:

(a)   In the case of hepatitis B and HCWs, the main aim of vaccination is for the protection of the vaccinated HCWs *themselves* against hepatitis B. However, for a small group of HCWs, the fact that they are immune to hepatitis B is also protective for their patients. These are the HCWs who carry out *exposure-prone procedures* (EPP), such as surgeons and midwives, where there might be a risk of infecting patients from these procedures. In this context, the vaccination program usually consists in giving the HCW a full course of hepatitis B vaccine, followed by a blood sample to check whether that HCW has developed adequate immunity to hepatitis B, that is, has a good enough level of hepatitis B antibodies. When this is the case, the HCW can be reassured that she is protected from acquiring hepatitis B infection, for example from an infected patient. However, she should still work in a safe manner to avoid being exposed to blood-borne viruses, as there is no vaccination against HIV and hepatitis C, for example. If she has attained adequate immunity to hepatitis B, then she is unlikely to be infected with hepatitis B (as long as she remains immuno-competent). If she were a surgeon or midwife undertaking EPPs, then the patients benefit from her immunity as they would not be put at risk of contracting hepatitis B through her. However, if she did not develop hepatitis B antibodies, she would normally have a repeat course of vaccination. She would also likely be tested for chronic hepatitis infection, as this is one of the reasons for not responding to vaccination. If she were a carrier, there is the possibility of treatment, maybe by a hepatologist or virologist. In the meantime, if she were deemed to be an infection risk (monitoring of her antigen status, for example, would reflect this), then she would be barred from performing EPPs until her blood results indicated that she were safe to perform these. This type of protocol ensures that patients are not put at risk from EPPs performed by HCWs who are hepatitis B carriers and remain infectious.

Now let us turn to the *ethical concerns* that can arise out of a hepatitis B vaccination program. These will usually turn around the issue of informed consent, as with most vaccinations, and if consent is *not* given, whether this refusal needs to be balanced against any other ethical requirement(s). For the most part, hepatitis B vaccination is for the HCW's own benefit, so as long as the decision is properly informed, then the HCW should be able to exercise her autonomous decision to decline vaccination. However, although the HCW may feel willing to accept the risk of subsequently become infected with hepatitis B, say through a needlestick injury, should she be allowed to take that risk? To put this into perspective, there will be a number of HCWs who do complete their hepatitis B course, but do *not* achieve an adequate antibody response (that is, remain at risk of infection). In both cases, a risk assessment might be appropriate, to see if they would be putting themselves at too high a risk, for example, working with known hepatitis B patients. If the risk could not be adequately controlled, then they would be safer to work in lower risk areas. This is not usually unduly restrictive in most clinical settings.

The ethical evaluation is different if the HCW performs EPPs. Here we must take account of **patient safety**, which of course is of major importance both in healthcare and OH. The postvaccination hepatitis B antibody level confirming an adequate response means that the HCW should be safe from contracting hepatitis B in the long term, and therefore could not transmit the infection to patients through EPPs. Thus, patient safety is ensured. Such a hepatitis B vaccination program, with HCWs demonstrating an adequate antibody response, is usually mandated for HCWs carrying out EPPs for this reason. Although in theory, this duty to protect patients could be invoked if the HCW declined, in practice such HCWs are unlikely to decline. They are usually highly motivated to pursue a career as a surgeon or midwife, for example, and so hepatitis B is probably not the best example to explore the ethical tensions that *could* arise between HCW autonomy and patient safety. There will be more realistic examples from other vaccination programs, with which to explore such tensions, as we will see below.

(b) The next example is that of chickenpox (varicella) vaccination in HCWs. Chickenpox is typically a mild illness in healthy children but can be a severe one in adults. It can be even more serious in immunocompromised individuals, pregnant women and fetuses, and neonates. Therefore, HCWs working particularly with these groups of patients must be immune to varicella zoster virus (VZV), so that they cannot contract the infection and transmit it to patients. The primary purpose of a VZV vaccination program is for the benefit of patients, especially those at higher risk of severe illness and complications. There is also benefit to vaccinated HCWs, as they then become immune to VZV infections. Similar ethical (and practical) concerns arise if the HCW declines VZV vaccination, as we saw in the case of hepatitis B vaccination. The main ethical tensions are between HCW autonomy and patient protection. However, the group of HCWs may be wider in scope, as it involves **all** HCWs in clinical contact with patients, rather than the smaller group of HCWs involved in EPPs when we considered hepatitis B.

When a HCW declines VZV vaccination, we may question whether this is a fully informed choice, so we should explore concerns and beliefs, and provide appropriate information. This allows the HCW to exercise their more reflective or reasoned autonomy (see Chap. 3). HCWs also have a professional duty to protect patients, often reinforced by their professional bodies' codes of conduct. This should also be part of their reflection. However, if they still refuse vaccination, then we should act in accordance with their choice. Nonetheless, it would not be ethical either to put patients at risk of potential severe infections. So, we would advise their manager that a risk assessment would be required, on the basis that the HCW is not immune to VZV. This should usually exclude them from clinical contact with the most vulnerable and high-risk groups of patients. However, there may be clinical settings where patient groups are variable, such as accident and emergency departments, so relocation to less acute areas with no high-risk patients might be required. On the issue of confidentiality, a "fitness certificate" with only the relevant information and advice, that is, the HCW lacking VZV immunity and the need for an appropriate risk assessment, addressed to the manager (possibly with a copy to HR) would **not** breach confidentiality in my view. It would still be preferable to have the HCW's permission to disclose this, but if the HCW refused, then our duty to protect patients from a serious illness should take precedence.

(c) The last example in this section is that of rubella. We have already reviewed rubella in a population context in the "Vaccinations and Public Health ethics" section. We have seen how it is usually a mild illness in adults but it can cause serious harm to a fetus if the mother contracts the infection. Female HCWs *do* benefit from being vaccinated if they do not have immunity to rubella, for the protection of their future children. On the other hand, *male* HCWs would have **no** benefit to themselves from being vaccinated against rubella. Rubella vaccination of HCWs is primarily for the benefit of patients who are either pregnant or of child-bearing age to protect their fetus. In the population health context, we argued that the value of **solidarity** meant that males should accept vaccination even though it did not benefit them. In the healthcare context, this still applies, but more importantly, I would suggest, is the professional and moral obligation of HCWs to protect the health of patients. The harm to a fetus from rubella infection is so great that it far outweighs any of the minor and transient ill-effects of the vaccine. A HCW who declined rubella vaccination could in theory have the same risk assessment approach applied as with VZV. However, in practice I have never experienced a HCW refusing rubella vaccine and doubt whether there would be many such instances. It is usually considered a mandatory vaccine for those working in clinical areas, and justifiably so.

Health Care Workers and Flu Vaccination

Influenza (flu) vaccination for HCWs programs share many of the ethical features of those we have discussed above in the hepatitis B, chickenpox and rubella vaccination programs. However, I believe that the arguments are more nuanced and merit further exploration. This is mainly because the evidence for effectiveness of such programs remain equivocal at best, as we will see later.

Mandatory?

Influenza can be a serious infection, particularly in some patients, such as elderly patients or those with chronic respiratory conditions. The flu vaccine is given to HCWs *primarily* to protect patients, especially the elderly. There is some benefit to the vaccinated HCWs, but current evidence appears to show that household infections are a more important means of contracting flu than the patient to HCW route. There is also much variation in the effectiveness of the vaccine from year to year, depending on how well the vaccine being used matches the circulating flu virus antigenic make-up. This is an important factor, often cited by HCWs who choose to decline flu vaccination. Nonetheless, a major strategy of many hospitals and other healthcare providers to reduce the burden of this potentially serious disease in patients has been to vaccinate HCWs against flu. HCW flu vaccination uptake has traditionally been variable (sometimes very poor), so some hospitals, such as in North America, have made it **mandatory** for HCWs to be vaccinated against flu.

Can mandatory HCW flu vaccination be morally justified? We have seen from Public Health (PH) ethics that in some circumstances, "quasi-mandatory" approaches could be morally defensible. On the one hand, the types of examples that would lead to this conclusion, that is a highly contagious and severe infection such as smallpox, are not the same as flu. On the other hand, HCWs have a greater moral responsibility to protect the health of their patients than other members of a community would have. Indeed, for those that argue that mandatory flu vaccination of HCWs can be morally justified, the duty to **protect** the health and welfare of patients is a key argument.

Review of the Evidence

If HCW flu vaccination definitely protected patients, then there would probably be a compelling moral argument that this *should* be compulsory, and there would be no place for HCW voluntariness in getting vaccinated. How good is the evidence that such programs achieve the desired patient protection? In a nutshell, the evidence is, at best, very weak. Reviews of the evidence (such as Cochrane reviews) point to the poor quality of available studies, so no definite conclusion on the effectiveness of flu vaccination of HCWs preventing transmission to patients is achievable. There is of course, some intuition that such vaccination must have a degree of protective effect. Amongst the reasons why a protective effect has not been measurable so far (apart from the poor design of many studies), is the fact that flu can also be transmitted to patients from infected hospital visitors and relatives, and other control measures such as hand hygiene may play an equally important role in limiting transmission.

Hierarchy of Control Measures

A thought-provoking review by O'Reilly et al (see Notes) reminds us of an important concept that we are very familiar with in OH practice: the *hierarchy of control measures*. Just as with any other hazard, focusing too much on one control measure (vaccinations) may in fact divert attention away from a more thought-through approach to preventing nosocomial flu infections. This may involve strategies such as limiting visitors during the seasonal flu season; excluding symptomatic staff and visitors; wearing of masks by some patients, visitors and staff; and especially emphasizing the importance of handwashing. There is a place for HCW flu vaccination as part of this overall strategy, but they point out that this will **not** completely prevent transmission on its own, even less so in seasons where there is mismatch between the vaccine and circulating strains.

Given the important, but limited, role that HCW flu vaccination can play in the prevention of flu nosocomial infections, do we think that making this vaccination mandatory for HCWs is morally justifiable? I think on current evidence, it is not. If we are serious about evidence-based medicine, then this is the approach we should take. An overall strategy taking account of all significant control measures, of which HCW vaccination would be one, would be my preferred approach. HCWs should be reminded of their duty to protect patients, but if this was within a framework where they **participate** in the control of flu transmission, I believe this would likely lead to *greater* patient protection.

Conclusion

Vaccinations are an important activity in OH practice and reviewing this topic also highlights some interesting ethical points. It reminds us of the importance of *informed consent*, as we are carrying out an intervention. Respect for autonomy of the worker needs to be balanced against the protection of others. In population health vaccination programs, the value of *solidarity* is often invoked as a reason to override individual autonomy if there is a threat of harm to other members of the community. In OH practice, it is often the worker's (usually HCW's) *professional duty* to protect the health of their patients that usually takes precedence. However, the example of HCW flu vaccinations highlights the importance of taking account of the evidence base in deciding to what extent patients are protected by the vaccination. In that example, I have suggested that mandatory flu vaccinations are **not** supported by current evidence. This may change as better-quality studies become available. Nonetheless, a strategy that addresses all the modes of transmission, seeks to control them *and* involves HCWs in participating in all elements of this strategy (vaccination being part of this) is likely to reduce the need for employers to be coercive with regard HCW flu vaccination. This may reduce ethical tensions and may also better protect patients.

Conclusion

Chapter 9
Conclusions

In this concluding chapter, I discuss the possibility of formulating a framework for OH ethics; share with you an ethical reflection tool for OH, with a worked example; think about what the future of OH could mean for OH ethics; and leave you with some final thoughts.

A Framework for OH Ethics?

Do we have a framework for OH ethics? It seems to me that this is something of a Holy Grail, and I do not claim to have achieved it in this book. First, let me clarify what I mean by "a framework for OH ethics". By this, I mean a "systematic approach which would guide us to the correct ethical choices in our OH practice". One problem, of course, is that often, there is no one single "correct" ethical choice. This may depend on the context and factors we need to weigh up and then make the best judgement we can. The other problem is that we do not have a *systematic* approach to resolving our ethical conflicts.

Several authors have proposed an approach (with minor variations) which I have found useful and have taught this to my students for many years. This is based on the four ethical principles of beneficence, non-maleficence, autonomy and justice. First, the relevant principles in the case would be identified. The second phase is to identify the relevant stakeholders, including the worker, employer and others. The third part is to weigh up the relative benefit or detriment that each stakeholder would have when one of the conflicting ethical principles is chosen over another. There is much merit in the simplicity of this approach to the ethical analysis of many OH practical problems.

However, the downside of such a simple approach is that one could argue that it does not always capture all the elements we need for a full ethical analysis, especially in more demanding and ethically complex cases. Some authors point out that deontological aspects may not be adequately captured by such existing models. I agree with them. We have professional, regulatory and legal requirements that may

© Springer Nature Switzerland AG 2020
J. Tamin, *Occupational Health Ethics*,
https://doi.org/10.1007/978-3-030-47283-2_9

not be given sufficient weight if these are not explicitly articulated within the model or framework. I have special concerns that the **dual obligations** that lie at the heart of all our OH interactions are not made explicit in the simple models. Similarly, it can be pointed out that moral obligations arising from a human rights discourse may not be adequately highlighted; for example, the right to have own's privacy respected. I realize that one could make a case for one to be reminded of this right to *privacy* through the principle of *autonomy*. However, autonomy and privacy are not the same thing, and further ethical problems can arise from conflating these two concepts. Furthermore, one can lose the benefit of examining moral problems through the lens of consequences, that is, *consequentialist* approaches are not applied in these simple models.

If we do develop a framework for OH ethics, I believe that in addition to the above comments (about sufficiently highlighting duties, rights and consequences), we should make our **dual obligations** a central feature of this framework. Many of the ethical problems that are special (if not unique) to OH arise from such obligations to different parties at the same time. I think we should also make the primary aim of OH (the **protection of workers' health** at work) another important feature of this ethics framework. Our aim to protect workers' health should act as a bearing for our moral compass, to guide us when arguments on both sides of an ethical argument or analysis are finely balanced. Although I have not developed such a framework, I would now like to share with you an ethical reflective tool which contains some of the features I have just mentioned.

Learning from Experience: Ethical Reflection

There are probably few more powerful ways of learning than through our own experience. Learning about ethics is no different. We need some awareness of ethical approaches and theories, but when we apply these to our **own** problem cases, we can develop much greater insight and understanding about how to resolve the ethical conflicts in our OH practice. So, if we spend time reflecting on cases where we have encountered ethical problems and if possible, share our reflections with peers, then we will continually learn from those experiences. For those who would like to document their reflections, I will describe a tool that I use for this purpose, which I have named "ERATOH".

ERATOH (Ethics Reflection and Audit Tool in Occupational Health)

I would like to share this reflection tool with you. There are such tools in clinical practice, but the ones I have tried deal with issues, for example, as deciding on treatment choices or involving the patient's relatives in difficult decisions such as at the end of life, which we do not routinely face in OH practice. Just as importantly, the clinical tools do not highlight the *dual obligations* that we owe to the worker and the employer. I have therefore developed this tool with the help of other members of my audit group, namely NWAG (North West Audit Group). They helped me pilot various iterations, and we currently use the version I have included at Appendix 4. If you find this helpful, feel free to use it, and even adapt it to better suit the context of your OH practice if you wish.

Such a tool is intended to act as an *aide-memoire*, a reminder of the important ethical duties and obligations that can come into play when we are faced with a difficult situation or decision in our practice.

The first question we must ask ourselves is: in which OH role am I operating in here? Is it in the *quasi-therapeutic* or the *independent* role (as explained in Chap. 2)? I think we are likely to be in the quasi-therapeutic role most of the time, but in pension ill-health retirement assessments and pre-employments assessments, we are usually in the independent role. You will recall that we have clear fiduciary obligations in the quasi-therapeutic role, but these are different in the independent role.

The table is organized into five columns (1–5) and five rows (A–E). The five columns are as follows: 1. Ethical considerations; 2. Worker; 3. Area of Practice or Issues; 4. Employer; and 5. Others (meaning other stakeholders). Under the "ethical considerations" column, the five rows are headlined as: A. Dual obligations of OH professional; B. Autonomy; C. Privacy/confidentiality; D. Non-maleficence/beneficence/justice/fairness; E. Summary/self-reflection. The fact that "Protection of worker health" is mentioned twice in the column serves to remind us that this is one of our primary objectives. Our "dual obligations" are also listed twice, to remind us of this key feature of our ethical obligations. Also, note that not all ethical considerations are necessarily listed in this column only. For example, "consequences" (relevant to consequentialist moral theories) appears in column 3, and "solidarity" is mentioned in column 5. To my mind, as long as their being mentioned helps you remember which of the ethical considerations might be relevant in the case you are analyzing, then it does not strictly matter at which point you are reminded of these points. So, if you do decide to use this or a similar template for your ethical reflection, feel free to re-arrange where the ethics "prompts" appear in this matrix and add or remove prompts to better suit your context.

In order to help you use this or your own modified template, I will continue by explaining why I have arranged the ERATOH template in this way. The first column lists some of the important ethical considerations. As this is an *ethics* reflective tool, this is reasonably intuitive. However, as OH practitioners, we may well be drawn first to the *third* column, as this is about the *practical* area or issue about the case we are reflecting on. The third column deals with the issues we usually think about in OH cases: are there problems with the diagnosis, effects on the worker's work capacity, communication issues or other conflicting interests? Could there be further consequences arising out of this case, depending on our advice, actions etc.? I have inserted this third column between those of the *worker* (second column) and the *employer* (fourth column) because all the OH issues will necessarily involve the worker, or the employer, or both. We often need to balance these interests (sometimes divergent), as well as those that arise from the fifth column ("other stakeholders").

If we now have a look at each row in turn. The first row has as its area of practice the **"diagnosis"** or the problem. Whatever the problem might be, the first column reminds us of our *dual obligations* to both the worker and the employer, and in addition, that it is important to gain the *trust* of both parties. With regards to the employer, there may be some specific questions he wishes us to address when we make our assessment. When we see the worker, we may need to clarify the issue, maybe the diagnosis or the clinical situation. This is not necessarily a problem and I expect most of such consultations not to raise undue ethical or professional concerns. However, here we are looking at cases that *have* caused us some moral unease, and we are looking at possible sources of such moral discomfort in this reflective approach. Whether the worker trusts us with his sensitive information may partly depend on whether he trusts the employer, which is why I mentioned the organizational values (or culture) in column 4. For example, if the employer is known to be supportive in providing necessary adjustments and so on, the worker may be more relaxed (and trusting) at the OH consultation than if the employer usually dismissed those with health problems. Although such factors may be beyond our control, they do frame the actual interactions we have with workers and the employer, which may sometimes be the source of the ethical tensions.

The area of practice of interest in the second row relates to the worker's **work capacity**, whether through his health being affected by workplace hazards, or whether the worker's health status has an effect on his ability to work. As previously mentioned, one of our main aims is to protect the health of the worker, especially from workplace hazards, so this should be uppermost in our mind (and appears in the first column). However, arguably the main ethical interest in this row is **autonomy**. This is relevant here at so many different levels. For example, a worker's *consent* (which is based on respect for his autonomy) is required before he can be assessed. Even his health protection (based on beneficence, with its overtones of paternalism—see Chap. 7) must be balanced with respecting his autonomy if he decides he would still rather risk his health (maybe rather than the possibility of losing his job). For consent to be valid, he must *understand* the information relating to the assessment and whether he decides to *accept* our advice or not is also an expression of his autonomy. From the employer and other stakeholder's perspective, if that worker's decision could put other parties at risk of harm, then his autonomy can be overridden. Furthermore, there may be legal standards or regulations (that is, duty-based demands) that an OH professional needs to adhere to that conflict with that worker's preferences, and the OH professional needs to resolve these conflicting ethical demands. On other occasions, ethical tensions can arise because of the *employer*. For example, a worker might be able continue working with appropriate *adjustments* in place, but the employer is unwillingly to provide or implement such adjustments. Sometimes this can be frustrating for OH professionals, but we need to learn to cope with such situations. Peer support and reflecting on difficult experiences in our practice may help us.

The third area of practice is that of **communication** (to both worker and employer, as well as others on occasion). This matches well with the ethical considerations of *privacy* and *confidentiality* (Chap. 4). However, what makes such communication more ethically complex in OH are our dual obligations and our primary duty to protect worker health, so we are again reminded of these in the first column. As mentioned in Chap. 6, as OH professionals, we are heavily involved in communicating to workers, managers and others, so this may well be a source of ethical conflict. The scenarios in Chap. 6 have illustrated the difficult balance between keeping worker information confidential *and* providing the employer with sufficient information. One or other party may disagree with our choice of where the balance ought to be in a particular situation. They may complain that we have disclosed either too much information (usually the worker) or too little information (usually the employer). These are matters for constant review and reflection. Furthermore, although we aim to protect the confidentiality of worker information, we may breach that confidentiality if others might be harmed as a result of *not* disclosing relevant information. We should make this clear in our advice to the worker at the start of the consultation. We normally require the worker's *permission to disclose* information in a report to the employer, but this requirement may not be absolute, for example, in situations of an independent assessment for a pension IHR report. Such exceptions may be further sources of ethical tensions and disagreements. On the other hand, the employer may also be frustrated with the need for the worker to give his permission to disclose a report and may not always understand our ethical constraints.

The next row is intended to be a "catch-all" for any issues or sense of moral unease that have not been captured by the previous rows. Why do we find this case or situation to be a problem? Does this stem from our duty to the worker? Duty to the employer? Our dual obligations? Do our moral duties of non-maleficence, beneficence or justice come into conflict, either with each other or with the previous ones we considered, such as autonomy and confidentiality? Do the possible consequences of our action (or inaction) cause us some concern? Do we feel a sense of injustice, at individual or systemic level? Are we able to do anything about this? This row also gives us an opportunity to reflect on wider issues that may be of concern to us, such as the impact of this OH situation on others: in the workers' families or their communities.

The last row is our summary of the salient issues that we wish to reflect on, and to discuss with peers if we have this opportunity. This is essential if we are to learn from experience, especially from our difficult cases. Now, with the benefit of hindsight, we may decide we might have done things differently. But the aim is not to feel guilt-ridden or inadequate. More often than not, the ethical tensions that need to be balanced are quite nuanced, and a "right" or "wrong" solution is often not possible. So, our aim should be to do the best we can in the circumstances, reflect on the experience, and hopefully do better (ethically) on the next occasion.

I will next describe a worked example of ERATOH, using the case of Ernie (from Chap. 6). I hope that by describing its use in this way, you will have a better understanding of how this reflective tool can be applied in your practice if you so wish.

An Example of Using ERATOH

The example at Appendix 5 uses an earlier iteration of ERATOH, previously called "ERATOM" (Ethics Reflection and Audit Tool for Occupational Medicine). As mentioned above, I will be using the case of Ernie (Chap. 6, case vignette (iv)). In this worked example, I had used a highlighter pen to identify those elements of the template I felt were more relevant to this case, but you can choose whatever approach you prefer, for example, underlining or circling relevant phrases in any boxes that you think will help you identify the issues you want to analyze and reflect on.

Ernie is a 45-year old supervisor in a chemical manufacturing company. Although he has been referred by his manager to see me (as opposed to seeing me as a self-referral; The distinctions are explained in Chap. 6), I would describe the relationship between Ernie and me as a *quasi-therapeutic* one, rather than an independent one. As you recall, this means that the fiduciary obligations that exist in the usual therapeutic healthcare professional-patient relationship are also present here. In Chap. 6, we focused on ethical issues that arose in the writing of a report to his manager. Here, although the ethical difficulties around communication and fitness for work remain the keys ones, the reflective tool allows us to think of broader ethical issues as well. For example, I listed the "neighboring community" as one of the possible stakeholders here. This is because Ernie works in a chemical plant, and it is possible for example, that if he collapsed while he was performing a safety critical task, this could lead to an explosion or the release of noxious fumes, which would affect the community. As we will see later, this is then included amongst the possible concerns we must balance when we are evaluating Ernie's fitness for work.

If we now look at the *problem* for which his manager referred him: this was a fall from a ladder. The manager is not aware of the preceding dizziness experienced by Ernie. There is uncertainty about the exact diagnosis, which could include Ernie's postural hypotension or his poorly controlled diabetes. It would be helpful to have more information from his GP (general practitioner) in due course, probably after Ernie has been evaluated by a specialist (possibly diabetologist). However, at this stage his GP will probably not be in possession of sufficient information to further clarify Ernie's clinical situation and give us an idea of his likely prognosis with appropriate treatment. With Ernie's permission, you could write a letter to his GP explaining your understanding of the situation and suggest a specialist referral (depending on your local circumstances and practice). Alternatively, Ernie could make an appointment with his GP and explain the situation himself. The way I approached Ernie's problem with him (and his wife) made it likely that I had gained Ernie's trust (which is especially important in a quasi-therapeutic relationship). However, I must not forget that I also have a duty to the employer. I noted that the manager only asked questions about fitness for work (FFW) and not about the possible causation of the fall. One of the difficult ethical issues I face is whether I should address the latter in my report to the manager, but we will look at this again when examining the issues around work capacity and communication (see below). In this example, I have not highlighted "organizational values", mainly because I was not sufficiently familiar with this employer to know what they were. Ernie himself was anxious that if the employer knew he had experienced dizziness and that this led to the fall, he might have the payment for physiotherapy stopped. He was also worried that if he not found to be fit for all his duties in due course, that he might be dismissed. Of course, his fears might be unfounded, but I could not guess whether the employer would be supportive and make any long-term adjustments to his job if required, or whether he would indeed dismiss Ernie. To the employer's credit, they were paying for the physiotherapy treatment, but I did not know whether this was through purely altruistic motives, or whether this was because of insurance or such purposes. At the time, I thought that I was neutral on whether the employer was supportive or not, but with hindsight (and discussion with peers) it is possible that I have given too much weight to Ernie's worries in my ethical analysis.

We next move to the reason for the management referral: Ernie's *work capacity*. His duties are described as being 80% non-physical (supervisory, administrative and control room work) and 20% physical. The plant is automated, and he spends most of his time in the control room, overseeing other workers. When there are fewer staff (mainly night and week-end shifts), he might need to do some physical work such as climbing ladders to do visual checks (of the gauges on vessels) and moving heavy pipes, connecting and disconnecting them to different vessels. However, as a supervisor, he does have the discretion as to who performs the physical work, and in the last few years he has rarely done much physical work, unless the staffing levels were very low or the workers on a shift were not sufficiently trained to do a particular task. This is in a chemical factory, where if things go wrong, there is a potential for disasters such as fires, explosions and toxic emissions into the atmosphere, which could affect workers and the neighboring community. Therefore, we should keep such H&S (Health and Safety) concerns in mind when assessing Ernie's fitness for work. We must also make Ernie aware of this, and that if there were risks to other individuals or the community, we might need to disclose information even without his permission, as part of the consenting process for me to carry out this work capacity assessment. Ernie understood the process and gave his informed consent for the assessment. Obtaining his consent in this way reflects our respect for Ernie's autonomy. In this case, they were no additional OH standards that needed to be applied, for example, had he been an emergency responder or a driver (where his dizziness could have been a bar to such roles). The need to apply such standards might then have been in conflict with his autonomy (that is, with his wish to continue working). However, we should adhere to accepted standards (usually evidence-based) as these are often designed to also protect the H&S of others (hence, non-maleficence) which would take precedence in such circumstances. I mention this here as a reminder, although such issues did not arise in Ernie's case.

The next practical consideration is that of *communication*. This links quite logically with the ethical requirements of *privacy* and *confidentiality*. But it also highlights our *dual obligations* in this area: The duty of confidentiality we owe Ernie must be balanced with our duty to the employer by giving his manager relevant information in our report. From Ernie's perspective, in addition to the report to his manager, there will be communications with his GP about his diabetic control and postural hypotension, and these will need to be with his permission. In this example, Ernie does give his permission for me to write to both his GP and his manager, so no ethical issues arise from tis. However, what I do and do *not* disclose in this management referral report are at the **center** of the ethical difficulties (as I experienced them) of this case. I have already discussed (in Chap. 6, case vignette (iv)) the problem of disclosing or not disclosing the dizziness symptoms to the manager, arguing that the question of causation (of Ernie's fall) had not been asked in the referral letter, so this allowed me not to address this issue, at least in the initial report. If you accept my position on this, then the report is fairly straightforward: it will detail advice on current and (near) future fitness for work; for longer term work capacity advice, Ernie would need to be reviewed and probably further information obtained from his GP and/or his specialist. However, if you do not agree with me not disclosing causation in this initial report, then you may feel that I haven't discharged my duty to the employer adequately. I understand such reservations about my approach and will look at this again in the next paragraph.

As I explained when describing Appendix 4, row D is the "catch all" section of the template, to allow us to re-consider any unresolved ethical issues or those not captured by the previous rows. It also allows us to think of other ethical duties or values not previously mentioned above, that may be relevant in this case. So, although my primary ethical concern in this case was whether I ought to disclose to his manager that Ernie was suffering from dizziness at times when he exerted himself, and this likely caused his fall from the ladder, I should not forget other factors at play, which may influence my ethical analysis. For example, if his symptoms could put other workers or the neighboring community at risk for example, if they could lead to a fire or explosion (given the chemical environment he worked in), then this risk would sway me to disclose the necessary information to prevent this from happening. I also owe Ernie a duty to protect his health (as this is the primary OH aim), so if my advice put him at risk of a further fall from heights, I would be failing Ernie in this duty. Nonetheless, in the scenario I have described, the likelihood of harm to himself or others is probably not significant, as he would be returning to administrative and supervisory duties, where he did not experience these symptoms. He would also have further evaluations (by his GP, specialist and myself) before he returned to more physically demanding duties, if he ever returned to these at all. Although Ernie expressed concerns about his employer withdrawing payment for physiotherapy, and even sacking him if he was not fully fit, I do not know whether he would really be treated in this way by his employer. Some employers might be very supportive and accommodate his limitations in the long term even if he did not become fit enough for physically demanding work. Other employers might insist that he had to be fit for all the duties in his job description as written, although in practice he had being doing less than the stipulated 20% physical work for several years. The latter type of employer might indeed terminate his contract if he were not found to be fit for all his duties. I have experience of both types of employers and you probably have as well.

You could point out that I have accepted Ernie's expressed concerns in an uncritical way. I would have to agree with you. But on the other hand, would I have been right to ignore his concerns and inform the employer that Ernie had experienced dizziness which could have led to his fall from the ladder? I do not think there is an easy answer either way.

The last row is where you would summarize your thoughts and reflect on the issues you highlight. This allows you to articulate your reasoning in support of the outcome and/or your preferred outcome on ethical grounds, now with the benefit of hindsight. You can also note any learning points and any different approaches you might take if faced with a similar situation in future. In addition, I use this ERATOH template as a basis for peer discussion in my audit group. In this case, most of my group felt that they would also not have disclosed Ernie's dizziness in the first report to the manager, but this was not a uniform view. Indeed, two of our group felt strongly that the employer was entitled to know this important fact. I accept that I was probably failing in my duty of veracity to the employer, but on balance I feel that such disclosure would probably have done more harm than good at that time (especially to Ernie).

Reflection and peer-group discussions are useful learning methods, but they do not always provide easy answers to difficult cases!

The Future?

In this section, I would like to first briefly consider future developments in OH and how these may affect OH ethics. I say *briefly* because other authors have adequately covered these topics, so I will merely highlight some of their findings. However, I *would* like to discuss a little more how these changes might affect a framework for OH ethics if (or when) we have one.

Those authors who have commented on the future of OH often point out the changing nature of work, which includes more precarious temporary and part-time work, remote and home-based work, older and migrant workers, as well as the advances in science and technology. Other significant changes are said to be the increasing global nature of the economy and more enterprises signing up to the concepts of *corporate social responsibility* and *sustainability*. It is argued in a recent report that the latter concepts widen the role of OH, going beyond physical health, to include a broader range of interests, such as the mental health of workers and social aspects of workers' lives.

So, how would a framework for OH ethics address such a broad range of interests? How would we develop a *corpus* of ethics to cope not only with the existing challenges in OH ethics, but also with those future challenges?

My suggestion is that this framework would consist of a **core** of OH ethical principles, values and approaches, and the flexibility to cope with a changing and wider scope for OH would be provided by additional **modules** to be used in the appropriate contexts, including the newer and emerging ones.

The *core* of this framework would be guided by the principles enunciated in ICOH's International Code of Ethics, with a special focus on our primary aim: the protection of worker health. The theoretical underpinning would be provided by the principlism approach (autonomy, beneficence, non-maleficence and justice), as well as relevant elements of duty-based, rights-based and consequentialist approaches. Last, but not least, it would take proper account of our *dual obligations* in all situations of ethical conflict.

As for the *modules*, these would be context-dependent and would need to be developed using specific ethical tools and approaches that would help to analyze the ethical problems that arise in each context. For example, if we were concerned about issues of social responsibility, then ethical approaches relevant to social justice, such as solidarity and possibly the *capability approach* (see Chap. 5) would be helpful. If we were dealing with issues arising from globalization and wondered about culturally-sensitive ethical norms, then we might need to draw on ethical approaches that emanate from different cultural and religious traditions. One can imagine any such relevant ethics modules could, when required in a certain context, be "bolted on" to the core OH ethics module which would remain central to this framework. I believe this would then provide us with the flexibility to meet future ethical challenges with the appropriate ethical tools and approaches.

Concluding Remarks

This book has been written primarily for OH practitioners. So, I have had as my focus those elements of ethical theory that might be useful in better understanding OH ethical issues that commonly arise in their practice.

In this chapter, I have described an ethical reflective tool and discussed what a comprehensive framework for OH ethics might consist of. I believe both approaches would better equip OH professionals to deal with existing ethical challenges, but also those that may emerge in the future.

A particularly insightful managing director of a company I worked for, over thirty years ago, said to me: "Jacques, you are the conscience of this organization." Over the years, we argued from different perspectives. I would make the case for improved working conditions on health and safety grounds, and he would sometimes reject these proposals on affordability grounds. But we continued to have a deep respect for each other. I knew he would have listened carefully and would give proper weight to my advice.

I hope you will also have the opportunity and privilege to influence organizational behavior for the good of workers and those who aspire to work. An element of the skill-set of OH professionals is the understanding of ethical approaches and their applications in their practice. However, in some situations there are no easy answers and we should continue learning from such experiences. It also sometimes takes moral courage and integrity to stand up for the right courses of action when organizations do not want to hear your advice.

So, I leave you with some advice that I usually give to my students: "Follow your conscience, but make sure your conscience is well informed.

Appendix A

Tamin J. Models of Occupational Medicine Practice: An Approach to Understanding Moral Conflict in "Dual Obligation" Doctors. Medicine, Healthcare and Philosophy. 2013, 16(3), PP 499–506

Abstract In the United Kingdom (UK), ethical guidance for doctors assumes a therapeutic setting and a normal doctor-patient relationship. However, doctors with dual obligations may not always operate on the basis of these assumptions in all aspects of their role. In this paper, the situation of UK occupational physicians is described, and a set of models to characterise their different practices is proposed. The interaction between doctor and worker in each of these models is compared with the normal doctor-patient relationship, focusing on the different levels of trust required, the possible power imbalance and the fiduciary obligations that apply. This approach highlights discrepancies between what the UK General Medical Council guidance requires and what is required of a doctor in certain roles or functions. It is suggested that using this modelling approach could also help in clarifying the sources of moral conflict for other doctors with "dual obligations" in their various roles.

Keywords Occupational medicine models, Occupational physician, Doctor-patient relationship, Dual obligation, Moral conflict, Fiduciary obligations

Introduction

In 2009, the United Kingdom (UK) General Medical Council (GMC) updated its guidance to doctors on confidentiality,[1] with supplementary guidance,[2] including a section entitled "Disclosing information for insurance, employment and similar purposes",[3] which clearly applied to doctors with "dual obligations",[4] including occupational physicians (OPs). One of the requirements was for the doctor to "offer to show

---

[1] GMC (2009a).

[2] GMC (2009b).

[3] pp. 22–26.

[4] The GMC (2009b, p. 24) state that "dual obligations arise when a doctor works for or is contracted (such as) by a patient's employer, an insurance company, an agency assessing a claimant's entitlement to benefits, the armed forces". The British Medical Association (BMA) 2012, p. 649 describes these as "situations where doctors have clear obligations to a third party that can be in tension to the obligation to the patient".

© Springer Nature Switzerland AG 2020
J. Tamin, *Occupational Health Ethics*,
https://doi.org/10.1007/978-3-030-47283-2

your patient, or give them a copy of, any report you write about them for employment or insurance purposes before it is sent".[5] This provoked great consternation amongst OPs. Most had been used to offering a copy of their report to the worker at the same time as to the employer or pension fund manager. Having to offer the report to the worker before the commissioning party however, could have significant implications to the way they practised. The UK Faculty (FOM) and the Society (SOM) of Occupational Medicine issued a joint statement which reflected this unease[6]: "Publication of this (GMC) guidance has caused widespread concern among OPs about the practical difficulties associated with compliance and unintended consequences relating to the impact that it may have on the perceived impartiality of reports".[7] In practice, OPs and occupational health (OH) providers have since changed their processes and consent forms to address this.[8] However, I suggest that there is a more fundamental reason why such ethical guidance does not sit comfortably with OM practice. I aim to show that the very nature of the doctor-patient relationship (DPR) is sufficiently different in OM practice compared with the therapeutic setting, for the same ethical rules to be at times incongruent in the former context.

To achieve this aim, I will describe OM as it is practised in the UK, and propose a set of models distinguishing the different OP roles and facilitating clearer comparisons between the OP situation and the normal therapeutic DPR.

OM in the UK

OM is that branch of medicine that deals with the effects of work on health, and of health on work.[9] In the past, an OP[10] would have been mainly concerned with the effects of toxic hazards in the workplace on the health of workers, but as work environments in the UK and other developed countries have become increasingly better controlled and safer,[11] the emphasis has shifted to assessing whether workers meet the appropriate medical standards for their occupation, that is, their fitness for work. A UK survey reveals that 75% of OP working time is spent on attendance

---

[5]p. 23.

[6]For example, an applicant who had been found not to meet the medical criteria for an early pension release due to ill-health, could simply refuse consent for this report to be released, and seek a more favourable opinion at a later date from a different physician.

[7]FOM, SOM (2010).

[8]For example, most consent forms for disclosure of a report now offer the opportunity for the worker to read it 2 to 5 days prior to sending to the employer.

[9]It is also part of the wider discipline of OH, which also includes nurses and physiotherapists, as well as ergonomists and occupational hygienists.

[10]An OP is a registered medical practitioner who has undertaken specialist training and qualifications in OM.

[11]For example, in Centre for Workforce Intelligence (2010): "Industry has changed from a manufacturing to a service majority over the last 20 years and this trend may continue. The main hazards have changed from dust, heat, noise and vibration to workplace pressure".

and absence assessments (Suff 2007). Thus the majority of an OP's time is spent in consultations to which the worker would have been referred by his manager for advice on fitness for work, and in a number of these cases, whether the worker would meet a pension scheme's criteria for early retirement on the grounds of ill-health[12] (IHR).

There are several other features of OM in the UK which may have a bearing on the OPW interaction. Firstly, in the UK, OH departments do not provide treatment services, except for first aid. Secondly, although the National Health Service (NHS) provides this treatment service, it specifically does not provide a National *Occupational* Health Service, so OH is largely *not* state funded.[13] Thirdly, although OH is mainly employer funded, there is no legal obligation on employers to fund this,[14] which is a different situation to that in some other European countries.[15] Lastly, there has also been a growing trend for OH services to be outsourced from in-house services to external commercial providers.[16] These background factors in UK OH provision may also contribute to some of the particular tensions that can arise between employers, OH professionals, and workers. However, before I describe the OP-worker (OPW) interaction in this context, the normal doctor-patient relationship will first be discussed, as this may clarify any differences between the two types of interaction.

The Normal Doctor-Patient Relationship (DPR)

Trust is said to be "intrinsic"[17] to the DPR.[18] O'Neill (2002) has described the DPR as a "paradigm of a relationship of trust...It is a professional relationship that is supposed to be disinterested, long-lasting, intimate and trusting".[19] Similarly, Brazier and Lobjoit (1999) have commented: "Patients trust doctors, nurses and other health professionals with intimate details of their lives which they may even conceal from their families".[20]

---

[12]For example a survey reported in Ballard J (2011) found that 17% of OPs list "dealing with IHRs" amongst their top three priorities (p. 22).

[13]FOM (2010a, p. 7).

[14]However, there is a statutory requirement for health surveillance of workers working with certain chemicals, or exposed to certain physical or biological hazards, for example, The Control of Substances Hazardous to Health Regulations 2002 SI 2002/267, and The Control of Vibration at Work Regulations 2005 SI 2005/1093.

[15]See for example: WHO Regional Office for Europe (2002) at p. 3.

[16]See for example in: FOM (2010a, p. 3) para 4.

[17]For example, De Zulueta P (2007, p. 14).

[18]However, many authors point out that there is not a "single" DPR, and have proposed various models to describe the different types of DPR . See for example Szasz and Hollender (1956) and Emanuel and Emanuel (1992).

[19]p. 17.

[20]p. 187.

Although this paper aims to highlight the differences between OM and all therapeutic medicine, rather than specifically between OM and general practice,[21] the importance of the DPR in the GP context has been described as its "central distinguishing feature" by Rogers and Braunack-Mayer (2009),[22] so the differences in the nature of the relationships may be more obvious between OM and GP. They also suggest that "trust in one area need not extend to trust in other areas. A patient may trust the goodwill of their GP in terms of confidentiality, affability, honesty and the like, but may not trust their competence in some clinical areas."[23] Likewise, O'Neill (2002) felt that she "might trust (her) GP to diagnose and prescribe for a sore throat, but not for a heart attack."[24] She also pointed out that polls show that doctors and judges are far more trusted than politicians and journalists.[25] Patient trust also appears to be the salient feature of the DPR on which the regulatory authorities, in the UK at least, base their ethical guidance to doctors: "Patients must be able to trust doctors with their lives and health."[26]

Although there may be different degrees of trust involved in different contexts, and trust may be situation- or condition-specific (such as the diagnosis of a sore throat rather than of a heart attack) there seems to be little doubt that trust is an essential component of the normal DPR.

The central role of trust in the DPR has led some authors to advocate that this relationship is subject to a fiduciary principle.[27] However, although trust is a requirement for a fiduciary relationship, it is not in itself sufficient grounds to claim that a relationship is fiduciary in nature. The duties imposed on the fiduciary to the beneficiary or vulnerable party are largely due to the power imbalance between the two parties. Such a power imbalance is said by Kennedy (1996)[28] to be evident in the DPR:

> The doctor-patient relationship has special, perhaps unique, features. Principal among these is the very significant disequilibrium of power between the two parties. The patient is uniquely vulnerable, being not only ignorant of the expertise constituted by the practice of medicine but also, in most cases, ill and anxious or anxious about possibly being ill. By contrast, the doctor has expert knowledge.

---

[21] Also known as Family Medicine (FM), but "General Practice" is more commonly used in the UK. A definition of GP/FM by WONCA (2011), the World Organisation of Family Medicine, describes GPs as "personal doctors" (at p8). In the UK, the GP is usually the first point of medical contact for most patients, other than for accidents and some emergencies, refers to specialist or other health services where appropriate, and maintains a long term relationship with his patients.

[22] p. 2.

[23] p. 31.

[24] p. 9.

[25] p. 10. A recent poll commissioned by the BMA, Munn F (2011), also confirms that the public trusts doctors far more than politicians.

[26] GMC (2006).

[27] See for example: Dyer AR and Bloch S (1987) p. 15; and Brazier M and Lobjoit M (1999) p. 187.

[28] p. 111.

Brody (1992) has drawn attention to the importance of the doctor's *power* in the therapeutic relationship, breaking this power down[29] to Aesculapian power (deriving from the medical knowledge and skills), social power (doctors generally coming from socially and educationally privileged backgrounds), and charismatic power (he postulated that many drawn to medicine would have this). The Law Commission (1992) has summarised the duties that arise in fiduciary relationships,[30] and Bartlett (1997)[31] amended these for the doctor-patient context:

1. *Fiduciaries must avoid conflicts of interest, or indeed even possible conflicts of interest, with the vulnerable party. (The "no conflict" rule).*
2. *Fiduciaries must not profit from their position without prior disclosure to and authorisation from the vulnerable party. (The "no profit" rule).*
3. *The fiduciary owes a duty of undivided loyalty to the vulnerable party. (The "undivided loyalty" rule).*
4. *The fiduciary owes a duty of confidentiality to the vulnerable party. (The "duty of confidentiality").*

Bartlett, Grubb (1994) and Brazier and Lobjoit (1999) have all presented strong arguments in support of the fiduciary nature of the DPR, although Kennedy (1996)[32] objects to this mainly on the basis that it "entrenches the paternalism and power of the doctor".

OM Models

I propose three models to describe the current UK OP-worker (OPW) interactions, accepting that this may not be exhaustive.

(a) Model 1: The "quasi[33]-therapeutic" model

As mentioned previously, OH services do not provide treatment in the UK, except for first aid. Some argue that because some OH departments administer vaccinations (such as against hepatitis B in health care workers, or for business travel) or can refer workers for physiotherapy or counselling, these constitute some element of "treatment", or at least of clinical care. On the other hand, although truly "therapeutic" encounters may be not part of OM in the UK, there are instances where OPW interactions may come close to being indistinguishable from the traditional doctor-patient ones, especially where a worker self-refers to the OH service or to the OP for advice. Although the OP cannot prescribe or treat in this scenario, the

---

[29]p. 62.

[30]Para. 2.4.9.

[31]p. 198.

[32]pp. 131–132.

[33]As in "seeming to be something but not really so", Oxford Essential English Dictionary, Oxford University Press, 2011.

encounter is often similar to a therapeutic one, in terms of the doctor giving advice, and presumably the worker trusting this advice, having sought it in the first place, hence a "quasi-therapeutic" encounter.

(b) Model 2: The "independent[34] expert" model

This model describes work such as IHR applications,[35] where the OP assesses the evidence presented (including specialist reports and evidence of attempts at workplace adjustments) against the medical criteria of the pension scheme. It would have similarities with expert witness work that doctors of any speciality can carry for the courts. However, for IHR medical assessments, it is the submitted evidence rather than the individual that is being assessed, so the applicant does not even have to be present in person[36] at a "consultation". One would expect the same advice by the GMC given to UK expert witnesses to apply,[37] for example in terms of the requirement to be "honest, trustworthy, objective and impartial".[38] This makes it clear that the expert's position is to be unbiased. In contrast, in an adversarial legal system, a lawyer must "present his client's best case and draw the court's attention to the weaknesses of the opposing party".[39] Both set of ethical obligations, for the expert to be unbiased on the one hand, and for the lawyer to be biased[40] on the other, are clear and unequivocal (albeit with some qualification for the lawyer). One would like to believe that other doctors (in a non-expert role) are also bound to be objective, unbiased and impartial in their judgments and their advice, but clearly this could be in conflict with their "duty of undivided loyalty" to their patient. This leaves them in the uneasy position where their duties from the two sets of obligations can be in direct opposition to each other.[41]

(c) Model 3: The "impartial[42] doctor" model

---

[34] For example, the term "independent" is used in the title "Independent Registered Medical Practitioner" (IRMP) in the Local Government Pension Scheme (Benefits, Membership and Contributions) Regulations 2007. The IRMP signs the certificate including the following statement: "I have not previously advised, or given an opinion on, or otherwise been involved in this case, nor am I acting or have ever acted as the representative of the member, the scheme employer or any other party in relation to it". Similar terminology is used in some other public sector pension schemes, such as "IQMP" (Independent Qualified Medical Practitioner) for the Firefighters' Pension Scheme Order 1992.

[35] Other work that would fall in this category includes OPs sitting on Medical Appeal Boards for these pension schemes.

[36] For the NHS Pension Scheme, which is the largest in the UK, virtually all are done remotely.

[37] GMC (2008).

[38] Para. 14.

[39] Devaney (2012).

[40] However, he must not knowingly mislead the Court (Bar Council 2004, paragraph 302).

[41] It is beyond the scope of this paper to offer a solution to this situation, except to note this intrinsic tension in the therapeutic role. It is the aim of this paper however to show that the differences between a treating doctor and an OP are such that in some aspects of the OP role (as expert, or model 2), this ethical conflict should not exist.

[42] "Impartial" being defined as "not favouring one person or side more than another", Oxford Essential English Dictionary, Oxford University Press, 2011.

This model will be used to describe the majority[43] of OP work, which usually arises from referrals by managers, asking for advice on workers' fitness for work, or health aspects of attendance or performance problems. Although the FOM recognises the need for OPs to be impartial,[44] it does also stress that OPs, like other registered medical practitioners, have an ethical responsibility to put the interests of individual patients first. Thus a physician, learning of a health risk to a worker, has "a responsibility to protect the health of the employee, even if this is to the detriment of the employer".[45] In the context of a health risk from work, this is understandable. However, in the UK workplace stress and musculoskeletal problems have become the predominant occupational illnesses. These are often more multifactorial in causation, and it remains an OP's responsibility to advise on such matters. But what does "putting the interests of individual patients first" actually mean in such cases? The employer may argue with some justification that it is the role of the GP to put the interests of his patient first. So in the UK, where the employer pays for the OP's advice, if this were to be no different to that received from a worker's GP, then the employer might question the value of paying for an OP's advice at all. An example would be where a worker suffers from work-related stress, which he alleges is caused by his manager bullying him. A report from his GP, if one were obtained, would be heavily biased towards his patient.[46] However, in many cases, there are other factors that may be relevant, such as feedback on poor performance by the manager to the worker prior to the alleged bullying. The OP should have a more balanced account of the situation, and be able to recommend more objective approaches, such as the use of stress risk assessments[47] or workplace mediation. If the OP were also simply to "put the patient first" in such circumstances, there is a risk that UK employers would largely cease to fund OH services,[48] especially as only a small proportion of OH work is legally required.

OM Models and Moral Implications

In model 1 ("quasi-therapeutic"), the OPW interaction is the closest to that between a doctor and patient in a normal DPR. Although a worker may not need to trust

---

[43] 75% of their workload, as previously mentioned, from the survey reported in: Suff P (2007).

[44] "Occupational physicians also need to build good relationships with **managers**. Integrity, respect, good communication, and a focus on **impartial** (emphasis added) evidence-based medical advice are important elements in building a relationship of trust in which patients' health problems and health and safety issues can be discussed constructively", FOM (2010b) p. 12.

[45] FOM (2006) p. 4.

[46] This is not intended to be a criticism of the GP, as the latter is clearly expected to put his patient first, and in addition he would have only one side of the story.

[47] See for example http://www.hse.gov.uk/stress/standards/downloads.htm.

[48] One of the consequences would be that less OH would then be available to UK workers, arguably to their detriment, as they would have even less access to expert advice and diagnosis for work-related conditions.

Fig. A.1 Obligations to patients versus society in model 2 and treating doctors

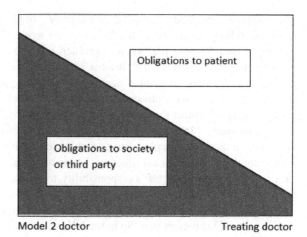

the OP with his "health and life", given that the OP will not carry out life-saving or other major interventions, he still needs to trust the OP to the extent that he is taking advice from the latter. Similarly, the power imbalance may be similar to that in the DPR, as the worker is generally in a position of knowing less than the OP about the health matter of concern. The main difference compared with the normal DPR is that fewer workers are likely to be as vulnerable as patients through pain and suffering, although some workers will seek help when they are distressed, especially if they have the facility to self-refer to the OH service. Given the similar levels of trust required and power imbalance in this model to the normal DPR, it is likely that the fiduciary obligations that arise in the normal DPR may also apply in model 1. Indeed, three of the four "central principles"[49] of a fiduciary relationship, namely the no conflict rule, the no profit rule, and the duty of confidentiality, seem appropriate in this context as well. On the other hand, the fiduciary's duty of "undivided loyalty" to the vulnerable party is less easy to support, given the OP's duty to the employer, and also to third parties if they could be harmed, for example. Although it could be argued that even in a therapeutic relationship, doctors also have obligations to third parties,[50] there is likely to be a difference of emphasis: the treating doctor usually puts his patient's interests first.[51] This is illustrated in Fig. A.1.

This figure illustrates the continuum between the two sets of obligations and the two extremes of the doctor role. However, for the purposes of this paper I will consider the treating doctor's obligations to be mainly towards the patient, and the model

---

[49] As described by Bartlett (1997).

[50] For example Gillon (1985), p. 158: "despite this acceptance (of obligations to society) doctors often talk and think as if they believe that they invariably give absolute moral priority to their patients over the moral demands of society". The GMC appear to reinforce this message: "you must make the care of your patient your first concern" (GMC 2006).

[51] In their role, one would find this partiality towards their patient acceptable, similar to Holm's (2011) arguments in support of such partiality in the context of public health care systems.

2 doctor to be mainly towards the third party, although this is clearly an oversimplification. In OM practice this different emphasis can be reflected in disagreements between the patient's treating doctor, such as the cardiologist of a train driver with a heart problem, and the OP who has to advise the employer on the risk assessment. The cardiologist may feel that the residual risk posed by his patient in terms of a sudden incapacitating event to be acceptable, but an employer or the public may take a different view.

In model 2 ("independent expert"), the OP acts as an expert assessor of evidence, for example for pension funds. There may be no direct contact with the worker (or applicant) in the UK, as the major public sector pension funds[52] use systems which involve the OP usually only reviewing the submitted evidence, and then presenting their advice or decision to the employer or pension fund managers. If there is any relationship at all between the OP and applicant, it would be, at best, an "arm's length" one, and therefore the level of trust required by the applicant would differ markedly from that expected of a doctor to whom he entrusts his life and health, or even accepts advice from. It would be limited to trusting that the OP has the appropriate training and qualifications to carry out this assessment, and will perform it competently and objectively. Such a level of trust bears little or no resemblance to that in the normal DPR, and would be more akin to that type of trust that we would have on a day to day basis in many individuals would provide us with a particular service, such as a surveyor assessing a building for electrical safety, and providing the required certificate.[53] Similarly, a power imbalance is less evident, or at least arguably less relevant. However, the OP is still in a some position of power,[54] as his advice or decision will determine whether the early release of the pension on ill-health grounds will proceed or not, and the applicant is in a position of vulnerability for the same reason. On the other hand, if there is no real relationship between the two parties, then the power imbalance seems to be an artificial consideration here. For example, although there is a clear power imbalance between a judge and a defendant when in court, this is not relevant in that context, and does not affect the validity of the process. The main reason for highlighting the power imbalance in the normal DPR (and other fiduciary relationships) is to provide the vulnerable party with some protection, by placing obligations on the fiduciary. In this model, the application of Bartlett's fiduciary principles to this context sits the least comfortably. One would not deny the need to avoid a conflict of interest or the OP profiting from his position, although it is difficult to see how the latter could do this, given the remoteness between the two parties. There could also be a need for some degree of confidentiality, although in practice most if not all the information will have been gathered by other parties beforehand. For example, the OP could find reference to

---

[52]This is the case for the largest fund, the NHS Pension Scheme. The other schemes may involve either a similar paper review, or a face-to-face assessment of the applicant.

[53]For example, if the property is to be let.

[54]On the other hand, the power imbalance can be reversed, for example when the applicant or his union representative threatens the OP with referral to the GMC and the courts if early ill-health retirement is not recommended.

distressing details in a psychiatric report about child abuse, and should be careful not to include such details in his report to the pension fund manager or trustees. However, such instances are rare, and a report for pension purposes will mainly concentrate on the applicant's ability to work, to perform certain tasks, and the likely permanence or otherwise of any health conditions and impairments. The fiduciary principle that would be completely incompatible with the OP's role would be the "duty of undivided loyalty", otherwise he could not give independent advice as required by the pension schemes.

Model 3 ("impartial doctor") represents the majority of OPW interactions in the UK, and reflects the need for OPs to be impartial in a "dual obligation" system. The types of interactions and obligations are more difficult to characterise, given the wide range of activities that are included here. However, that range can be illustrated by two examples[55] of activities in this model: on the one hand, for "health surveillance"[56] activities, the OP may be towards the right of the Fig. A.1 "model 2/treating doctor axis". That is, there is significant obligation towards the worker, as this activity concerns protecting workers' health from workplace agents.[57] On the other hand, for sickness absence referrals (the majority of OP work) the OP would be more to the left of that axis, as usually this is more for the employer's benefit. From a relationship perspective, model 3 is in the "middle ground"[58] between models 1 and 2, and the worker may be somewhat disappointed that the OP is not "taking his side". In the normal DPR, the importance of trust and the power imbalance in that relationship is very evident. It is not suggested that in this third model, trust or power imbalance play no part. Rather, it is likely that the nature and extent of any trust and power imbalance are different. As O'Neill points out, we can trust individuals in some matters but not others,[59] or to different extents. For example, in the DPR, patients should be able to "trust doctors with their lives and health".[60] This level of trust is not required from workers in the normal OH consultation. Indeed, it would be rather surprising if anyone expected such a level of trust. On the other hand, one would hope for some trust in the OP, for example of his competence at evaluating health and work issues (although some workers challenge this when the assessment results are not to their liking), and of his honesty and integrity (although this trust becomes less evident

---

[55] Although these examples serve to illustrate the different levels of obligations in model 3, the main aim of this paper is to demonstrate that at the extremes (i.e. models 1 and 2), the underpinning ethical reasons for doctors' obligations are different, so that the anomalies and conflicts arising in the ethical guidance are due to its being based on wrong assumptions.

[56] That is, monitoring workers' health from workplace exposures to chemical, physical or biological agents, under legislation such as mentioned at ref (14).

[57] However, this is also to a lesser extent for the benefit of employers, for example, in discharging their duties under health and safety legislation.

[58] But as seen from the examples, the middle ground is not a fixed point on the figure 1 "model 2/treating doctor axis", but will vary according to the type of activity, and maybe the context.

[59] O'Neill O (2002), where at p. 9 she gives the following examples: "I might trust a schoolteacher to teach my child arithmetic but not citizenship... I might trust my bank with my current account, but not my life savings".

[60] GMC (2006).

when increasing emphasis is placed on signed consent(s), and a worker reading the report before its issue). Similarly, in the normal DPR it is argued that the power imbalance arises partly from the patient being ill and more vulnerable than he would otherwise be, and partly from the doctor's power. In the OPW situation, the worker is often not ill, but may still be more vulnerable through lack of expert knowledge, which the OP will have. However, there are also situations where the power imbalance shifts in the opposite direction, for example, when workers attend with their union representatives who can be very knowledgeable on the relevant issues, or be coercive (such as threatening to refer the OP to the GMC) if the favourable outcome were not obtained for their member. Although such situations are relatively rare, they serve to illustrate that the power imbalance may not always be as one imagines it to be.[61]

OPs aim to be impartial whichever model they are operating in, as it is a requirement of their function. Nonetheless, it is a difficult balance to achieve in everyday practice.[62] In model 1, where the relationship may be close to the DPR, there is probably a greater risk that the OP could develop a closer affinity with the worker's views, although he may not recognise this himself. However, even in this model, if the outcome of that consultation were unwelcome by the worker, the OP is still not bound by a "duty of undivided loyalty". Indeed, the duty of undivided loyalty cannot be expected of the OP in any of the three models, although the incongruity of expecting such a duty in OPW interactions is most evident in model 2, where the independence of the OP is essential. If in the DPR, trust and power imbalance are of central importance in the analysis of that relationship, then it is suggested that in this third model, the emphasis should be on the *impartiality* of the OP. This need for impartiality can create tensions with the worker and the employer (and other stakeholders, such as "the public"[63]).

Other doctors with dual obligations, such as in sports, insurance[64] or military medicine, may also be in situations where some of their roles fit the normal DPR

---

[61]It is accepted that even in the DPR, a GP may occasionally feel threatened by his patient, and prescribe some medication or write a certificate, against his better judgment.

[62]These models are intended to be a description of current UK OM practice, rather than what it ought to be. It is accepted, for example, that if OH provision became state rather than employer funded, this would change the pressures arising from the employer-OP relationship. Alternatively, OPs could adopt a definite servant-master approach with employers, which arguably would make it clearer for all parties to understand the OP role(s). However, whether one of these, or other approaches were to be pursued, it would still take some time to come into effect. In the meantime, it is hoped that a clearer understanding of the different tensions, and why they arise, will help OPs in their practice, and regulators producing ethical guidance.

[63]For example, passengers and other members of the public, when a train driver suffers from epilepsy and does not want this to be disclosed by the OP.

[64]For example, Grubb (1994) p. 334, opines that the insurance medical context would not give rise to a fiduciary relationship: "One of the most important conditions for the (fiduciary) duty to arise is absent: an entrusting of power by the beneficiary which is to be exercised *only for his benefit.*" This condition is also absent in OM models 2 and 3, and presumably in some sports medicine and military medicine situations.

Table A.1 Trust, power imbalance and fiduciary obligations in the three OM models compared with normal DPR

	Normal DPR	Model 1 "quasi-therapeutic"	Model 2 "independent expert"	Model 3 "impartial doctor"
Trust	Very important	May be similar to normal DPR	Very limited	Limited. For example, that even in a non-therapeutic context, certain professional standards will apply
Power imbalance	Usually significant	May be similar to normal DPR	May not be relevant	Variable
Fiduciary obligations 1. No conflict (of interest) rule 2. No profit rule 3. Duty of undivided loyalty 4. Duty of confidentiality	Consistent with all four fiduciary central principles	May be similar to normal DPR, except for duty of "undivided loyalty"	Fiduciary obligation of "undivided loyalty" is totally incompatible as independence is essential	Limited fiduciary obligations

paradigm, but at other times be in roles where that paradigm does not apply.[65] In the latter cases, as with the OM situation, different ethical guidance for the situations that are similar to models 2 and 3 that recognises these differences may help to reduce or resolve moral conflicts.

This table summarises the main differences described above (Table A.1).

Conclusion

Ethical guidance for doctors is usually based on the assumption that a normal DPR exists. By using the modelling approach in OM, it becomes evident that not all OPW interactions fit this assumption. On the one hand, in model 1 the OPW interaction is close to the normal DPR, and therefore not surprisingly most of the ethical constraints in a normal DPR make sense in model 1. At the other extreme, when the interaction is

---

[65]It is envisaged that the equivalent of models 1 and 2 could be reasonably clearly established for other dual obligation disciplines, though they would be different to the OM models. For example, in sports medicine, model 1 would actually be therapeutic, and the arm's length model 2 arises for example during a pre-transfer medical assessment of a prospective team player. The middle ground, model 3, could arise for example when the team coach wanted a player recovering from injury to play possibly too early in an important match, and the club doctor had to advise.

very "arm's length" (model 2), most of the underlying assumptions used in the normal DPR are incorrect in that situation. The fiduciary obligation of undivided loyalty, for example, is incongruous if applied in a context where independence is essential. In model 2, the ethical requirement (by the GMC) for the OP to offer to show his report (of an independent assessment) to the applicant before submitting it to the employer or pension fund manager would be akin to a judge offering a defendant first sight of his judgment, and requiring the defendant's consent before delivering it. It would be helpful if regulators such as the GMC could make a distinction between these different situations, and adjust the guidance to reflect the reality of the different OM roles.

Acknowledgments I wish to thank Professor Søren Holm and Dr. Sarah Devaney for helpful comments and suggestions.

Conflicts of interest None.

References

Ballard J. 2011. *OH professional practice, Part 1: jobs, priorities, concerns, threats and opportunities*, Occupational Health [at Work], 8(1): 21–27.

Bar Council. 2004. *Code of Conduct*, 8th edition.

Bartlett P. 1997. *Doctors as fiduciaries: Equitable regulation of the doctor-patient relationship*, Med Law Rev, 5: 193–224.

British Medical Association. 2012. *Medical Ethics Today: The BMA's Handbook of Ethics and Law*, 3rd edition, London.

Brazier M and Lobjoit M. 1999. *Fiduciary Relationship: An Ethical Approach and a Legal Concept?* In Bennett R and Erin CA (Eds), *HIV and AIDS testing: Screening and Confidentiality*; Oxford University Press: 179–199.

Brody H. 1992. *The Healer's Power*, Yale University Press.

Centre for Workforce Intelligence. 2011. *Medical Specialty Workforce Factsheet: Occupational Medicine*, http://www.cfwi.org.uk/intelligence/cfwi-medical-factsheets/recommendation-for-occupational-medicine-training-2011.

Devaney S. 2012. *Balancing duties to the court and client: The removal of immunity from suit of expert witnesses*, Med Law Rev (forthcoming)

De Zulueta P. 2007. *Truth, trust and the doctor-patient relationship*, Primary Care Ethics, Radcliffe-Oxford: 1–24.

Dyer AR and Bloch S. 1987. *Informed consent and the psychiatric patient*, J Med Ethics, 13: 12–16.

Emanuel EJ and Emanuel LL. 1992. *Four models of the Physician-Patient Relationship*, JAMA, 267: 2221–6.

FOM. 2006. *Guidance on ethics for occupational physicians*, 6th edition, Royal College of Physicians, London.

FOM. 2010a. *Future directions for the occupational health care in the UK, A strategic overview*, http://www.facoccmed.ac.uk/library/docs/pp_natstrat.pdf.

FOM. 2010b. *Good Occupational Medical Practice*, Royal College of Physicians, London, http://www.facoccmed.ac.uk/library/docs/p_gomp2010.pdf.

FOM, SOM. 2010. *Joint statement to FOM & SOM Members, New GMC Guidance on Confidentiality 2009*.http://www.som.org.uk.

Gillon R. 1985. *Philosophical medical ethics*, John Wiley & Sons, Chichester.

GMC. 2006. *Good Medical Practice*, London.

GMC. 2008. *Acting as an expert witness: Supplementary guidance,* London.

GMC. 2009a. *Confidentiality*, London.

GMC. 2009b. *Confidentiality: Supplementary guidance,* London.

Grubb A. 1994. *The doctor as fiduciary*, in *Current Legal Problems* (Ed. Freeman MDA), University College London, 47 b: 311–3.

Holm S. 2011. *Can "Giving preference to my patients" be explained as a Role Related Duty in Public Health Care Systems?* Health Care Analysis, 19: 89–97.

Kennedy I. 1996. *The fiduciary relationship and its application to doctors and patients*, in *Wrongs and Remedies in the twenty-first century*, (Ed. Birks P), Oxford University Press: 111–140.

Law Commission. 1992. *Fiduciary Duties and Regulatory Rules*, Consultation Document 124, HMSO.

Munn F. 2 July 2011. *Public declares doctors the most trusted professionals*, BMA News Review: 2.

O'Neill O. 2002. *A Question of Trust, The BBC Reith Lectures 2002*, Cambridge University Press.

Rogers WA and Braunack-Mayer AJ. 2009. *Practical Ethics for General Practice*, 2nd edition, Oxford University Press.

Suff P. 2007. *Welcome to the working week (OH work survey)*, Occupational Health [at Work], 4, 3: 22–28.

Szasz TS and Hollender MH. 1956. *The basic models of the doctor-patient relationship*, AMA Archives of Internal Medicine, 97: 585–592.

WHO Regional Office for Europe. 2002. *Good practice in Occupational Health Services: A contribution to Workplace Health,*http://www.euro.who.int/__data/assets/pdf_file/0007/115486/E77650.pdf.

WONCA EUROPE (2011). The European definition of general practice/family medicine, accessed at http://www.woncaeurope.org/.

Appendix B

Tamin J. Mandatory Flu Vaccinations? Occupational Health at Work. 2016, 13(3), PP. 29–31

Reproduced with the kind permission of the editor of Occupational Health at Work.

Occupational physician Jacques Tamin believes that campaigns to improve uptake of influenza vaccine among healthcare workers should take account of current evidence and thus target only those caring for patients most vulnerable to the disease. Blanket vaccination of all healthcare workers is not morally justified.

According to Public Health England and NHS England: 'Every year, influenza vaccination is offered to NHS staff as a way to reduce the risk of staff contracting the virus and transmitting it to their patients.[66] In 2014/15, their 'flufighter' campaign achieved a vaccine uptake rate for frontline healthcare workers (HCWs) of 54.9%[67] and, despite the efforts of NHS occupational health (OH) departments, achieving the national target of 75%[68] seems extremely optimistic.

It could be argued that attempts to improve HCW uptake have so far not been very successful (although there are wide variations, with aggregated averages ranging from 42 to 76%[69]). In the US, when some healthcare organisations made influenza vaccination mandatory as a condition of employment, rates went up to over 98[70] and

---

[66] Public Health England. Healthcare worker vaccination: clinical evidence (updated October 2015). Flufighter: NHS England Publications Gateway Reference 04249. ohaw.co/2bRs9Zv (accessed 30.8.16).

[67] Public Health England. Seasonal influenza vaccine uptake amongst front line healthcare workers (HCWs) in England, Winter season 2014–2015. May 2015. PHE Publications. ohaw.co/2bITVE3 (accessed 30.8.16).

[68] Ibid p. 13.

[69] Public Health England. Seasonal influenza vaccine uptake amongst front line healthcare workers (HCWs) in England, Winter season 2014–2015. May 2015. PHE Publications. ohaw.co/2bITVE3 (accessed 30.8.16).

[70] Babcock HM, Gemeinhart N et al. Mandatory influenza vaccination of healthcare workers: Translating policy to practice. Clinical Infectious Diseases. 2010; 50: 459–464. https://doi.org/10.1086/650752.

© Springer Nature Switzerland AG 2020
J. Tamin, *Occupational Health Ethics*,
https://doi.org/10.1007/978-3-030-47283-2

99%.[71] Could we envisage a similar approach in the UK? And would we consider this to be morally justifiable?

A debate paper in the *British Medical Journal* (BMJ) supported mandatory influenza vaccination on the one hand,[72] and refuted it on ethical grounds on the other.[73] The paper in favour emphasised patient safety, and the fact that voluntary approaches did not achieve the target uptake rates. It also claimed that HCW vaccination reduced sickness absence. The authors against mandatory vaccination argued their position mainly on the basis of HCW autonomy, but also suggested that coercive approaches would alienate and demoralise the workforce.

In order to clarify the ethical arguments from both positions, it may be helpful to understand the ethical concepts that are more generally deployed in public health vaccination programmes.

Public Health Vaccination Programmes

For population health programmes, if sufficient members of their community are vaccinated, that community is protected through 'herd immunity'. However, if a purely voluntary system does not recruit the required numbers, would there ever be justification for overriding individual consent? That is, could it ever be morally justifiable to apply coercion or compulsion in order to achieve this wider benefit to society?

The Nuffield Council on Bioethics suggests that an ethical framework for public health needs to include values that emphasise the benefits to all members of society. Such an approach is often described as 'solidarity'. This value is central in 'the limitation on individual consent when it obstructs important general benefits.[74]

In deciding whether solidarity could prevail over individual consent, one would take into account the severity of the infection itself, whether prevention of transmission could be achieved in other ways, the effectiveness of the vaccine, and the incidence and severity of side effects of the vaccine. The consent—solidarity balance is therefore likely to vary for different vaccination programmes. The Nuffield Council 'identified two circumstances in which quasi-mandatory vaccination measures are more likely to be justified. First, for highly contagious and serious diseases, for example with characteristics similar to smallpox. Secondly, for disease eradication if the disease is serious and if eradication is within reach.[75]

---

[71] Parada JP, Koller M et al. No more Mr Nice Guy—implementation of mandatory seasonal influenza immunization for all personnel. BMC Proceedings 2011; 5 (Suppl. 6):276. https://doi.org/10.1186/1753-6561-5-S6-P276.

[72] Helms CM, Polgreen PM. Should influenza immunisation be mandatory for healthcare workers? Yes. BMJ 2008; 337: a2142. https://doi.org/10.1136/bmj.a2142.

[73] Isaacs D, Leask J. Should influenza immunisation be mandatory for healthcare workers? No. BMJ 2008; 337: a2140. https://doi.org/10.1136/bmj.a2140.

[74] Nuffield Council on Bioethics. Public health: ethical issues. London: 2007, at p. 23.

[75] Ibid p. 60.

At present, no truly compulsory public health vaccination programme exists. However, there are several examples worldwide of 'quasi-mandatory' programmes, where unvaccinated individuals cannot access some benefit, such as access to education. It has been argued that penalising children by denying them access to education is itself morally repugnant,[76] so a balance needs to be struck between the benefits of vaccination, and the harms of a quasi-mandatory approach, particularly from the sanctions that are used.

Influenza Vaccination of HCWs

The justification for influenza vaccination of HCWs is different. It does not seek to achieve herd immunity, but aims to protect vulnerable patients by preventing transmission from infected HCWs.

A recent review of the practicalities of influenza vaccination in an OH context concludes that 'while vaccination of HCWs is necessary, on its own it may not be sufficient to prevent nosocomial influenza infection, and a multidimensional approach is clearly required.[77] The authors advocate a risk management approach, including a comprehensive review of the control measures in place to prevent nosocomial influenza transmission. This approach resonates well with OH practice, where we are familiar with the hierarchy of controls, and a risk assessment methodology. For example, even if all HCWs are vaccinated against influenza, this would not stop transmission from visitors to patients, so control strategies need to take such factors into account.

In the BMJ debate paper, Isaacs and Leask argue that mandatory vaccination 'infringes civil liberty and autonomy.[78] Autonomy is also the main interest protected by the requirement of 'informed consent'.

However, if what we value in being autonomous is the right to self-determination, the ability to make choices that are aligned with our deeply held values and beliefs, then it could be argued that an individual HCW's autonomous choice should be that which would protect their patients. After all, should we not expect 'putting patients first' to be at the core of HCWs' values?

Furthermore, HCWs have a duty to protect the health of their patients, a duty that is embedded in their professional regulation, and it is what the public expects of them.

---

[76]Glover-Thomas N, Holm S. Compulsory vaccination. In: Stanton C, Devaney S et al., editors. Pioneering healthcare law: essays in honour of Margaret Brazier. Abingdon: Routledge, 2015, pp. 31–42.

[77]O'Reilly F, Dolan GP et al. Practical prevention of nosocomial influenza transmission, 'a hierarchical control' issue. Occupational Medicine 2015; 65: 696–700. https://doi.org/10.1093/occmed/kqv155.

[78]Isaacs D, Leask J. Should influenza immunisation be mandatory for healthcare workers? No. BMJ 2008; 337: a2140. https://doi.org/10.1136/bmj.a2140.

Why then do some HCWs—at present about 45% in the UK—ignore the calls to be vaccinated in order to protect their patients? Studies that have looked into this question give us a range of fairly similar reasons, including: doubts as to the efficacy of the current vaccine; fear of side effects; and not believing that being vaccinated would protect their patients. Factors that improve uptake include concerted educational efforts and ease of access to vaccination. One should acknowledge that some of these concerns are well founded. Vaccine effectiveness does vary seasonally, and depends on how well the vaccine and the circulating strain are matched. In addition, the evidence for patient protection resulting from HCW influenza vaccination is at best weak, and sometimes equivocal. There is some reported evidence that vaccinating HCWs working with highly vulnerable elderly populations in long-term care settings can be effective[79]; but this has been countered by a recent Cochrane review, which found little conclusive evidence of benefit.[80]

Returning to our consideration of an HCW's autonomous choice, the argument would then be as follows: even when we take into account their values (to protect patients) and professional duties, the only patients that vaccinated HCWs might conceivably protect—on grounds of their increased vulnerability to the disease— would be elderly patients in long-term care facilities. One might argue that HCWs who are in contact with such vulnerable patients *ought* to decide to be vaccinated, and this would be consistent with their autonomous choice, given their commitment to patient safety.

	OH Law
Advance notice	Introducing OH Law Online
New service for *Occupational Health [at work]* subscribers	Special loyalty discount for *Occupational Health [at Work]* subscribers Save £50 + VAT!
Gain CPD as you read, learn, research, discuss and reflect	

(continued)

---

[79]O'Reilly F, Dolan GP et al. Practical prevention of nosocomial influenza transmission, 'a hierarchical control' issue. Occupational Medicine 2015; 65: 696–700. https://doi.org/10.1093/occmed/kqv155.

[80]Thomas RE, Jefferson T, Lasserson TJ. Influenza vaccination for healthcare workers who care for people aged 60 or older living in long-term care institutions. Cochrane Database of Systematic Reviews 2016; 6: CD005187. https://doi.org/10.1002/14651858.CD005187.pub5.

(continued)

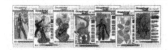	OH Law
From the Dec/Jan issue, *Occupational Health [at Work]* will feature a brand new continuing professional development (CPD) service for subscribers. Each issue will feature an article with additional CPD activity associated with it, and the new service will enable you to record CPD gained from reading *Occupational Health [at Work]*. We estimate that subscribers could easily gain up to 15 h of CPD a year from reading *Occupational Health [at Work]* and carrying out the CPD activities. Look out for the new CPD Personal Learning Zone in the next issue of *Occupational Health [at Work]*!	**OH Law Online** is the new online subscription service from The At Work Partnership—providing the latest information on occupational health law, and explaining the key areas and their implications for your work. **Find out more!** Visit www.ohlaw.uk to see the latest OH legal news. You'll find one section of the site—examining OH regulation and liability—is available FREE. Click on the "Find out more" button on the website for a link to this. Visit www.ohlaw.uk to browse our free content, to sign up for our free email newsletter and to subscribe today.

Smart Thinking

The mandatory influenza vaccination of *all* HCWs is not morally justifiable, given the current evidence on patient protection. I would go further and say that educational programmes aimed at all HCWs ought to be accurate and transparent, and should be honest about where the evidence is either good or weak with regard to patient protection. They should also acknowledge seasonal variations of vaccine efficacy. There are some personal benefits from being vaccinated, but these are a matter of personal choice. For example, there is no good evidence that it reduces HCWs' *occupational* influenza infections—the evidence is that *household* exposures are more relevant—or that it significantly reduces sickness absence.

On the other hand, I believe that a quasi-mandatory programme—i.e. making it a contractual requirement—could be justified for HCWs working with vulnerable elderly patients in long-term settings, if a voluntary approach does not achieve a sufficient uptake of vaccination. Quasi-mandatory HCW vaccination programmes have been implemented for other diseases where evidence for patient protection is felt to justify them. These include immunisation against measles and rubella, where the HCW who refuses vaccination is prohibited from working in contact with the relevant vulnerable patient group. But as OH practitioners would we be comfortable implementing such a quasi- mandatory influenza vaccination programme on the available evidence? Would consent be valid in such circumstances?

It may be a better use of resources, and therefore more ethical, to first target those HCWs who work with the vulnerable patient groups, using increased educational and awareness campaigns, rather than the current scattergun strategy, which has so far been of limited success.

I would suggest that NHS England's strategy of targeting *all* HCWs for flu vaccination is not justified on current evidence, and so a mandatory approach would be unethical. A more focused approach targeting the highest risk areas—that is, elderly patients in long-term settings—may achieve better uptake rates. If an educational and facilitative approach did not achieve these, then I argue that quasi-mandatory flu vaccination of this group of HCWs would be ethically justified.

Jacques Tamin is an occupational physician. He is an honorary senior lecturer at the Centre for Occupational and Environmental Health, University of Manchester. He has a PhD in bioethics and medical jurisprudence from the University of Manchester.

Conclusions

- The main objective for flu vaccination of healthcare workers is to protect patients
- The evidence that this strategy is effective is extremely limited
- It is argued that only healthcare workers working with elderly patients in long- term settings might be targeted on grounds of this group's increased vulnerability to the disease
- Quasi-mandatory flu vaccination of healthcare workers working with elderly patients in long-term settings could be ethical
- Mandatory flu vaccination of other healthcare workers would not be morally justifiable.

Appendix C
Transcript of Sandy Elder Award 2014 Presentation

Sandy Elder Award 2014

Occupational Health ethical confusion: could Public Health ethics help?[81]

Jacques Tamin

Centre for Occupational and Environmental Health, and Centre for Social Ethics and Policy, University of Manchester, UK

Acknowledgments I wish to thank the Sandy Elder Award for funding this project. I note that Sandy has been described as "a master of the theory and the practice of ethical communication in medical practice".[82] I therefore hope that he would have welcomed my small contribution in this area of interest.

Abstract There is evidence that UK occupational physicians are confused about some ethical issues, such as confidentiality and consent. There may be different reasons for this. One of these reasons might be that we serve communities of workers, as well as individual workers. There may therefore be some similarities between ethical issues in occupational medicine (OM) and public health (PH). This paper seeks to explore whether a consideration of PH ethical approaches may help reduce confusions that arise in OM ethics. In particular, the examples from PH of health data sharing and vaccination programmes are analysed, with reference to confidentiality and consent respectively. It concludes that there are some useful concepts that could be learnt from the PH examples, such as that of solidarity.

---

[81] This paper was presented at the Scottish SOM Spring 2016 Conference on the 28th April 2016.

[82] Macdonald EB, Symington IS and Soutar R. Alexander ("Sandy") Gordon Elder. *BMJ* 2007; **334**(7585):161.

© Springer Nature Switzerland AG 2020
J. Tamin, *Occupational Health Ethics*,
https://doi.org/10.1007/978-3-030-47283-2

Introduction

In the UK, there is "significant current variation between occupational physicians and uncertainty regarding best practice with regard to consent and confidentiality".[83] So, what could the cause of such uncertainty? It has been suggested that some of this confusion may arise from differences in the doctor-worker relationship itself,[84] and from the conflict between GMC guidance[85] and the law,[86] although there is some debate on the latter point.[87] However, it is possible that other factors also contribute to this confusion, such as the fact that the occupational health (OH) ethical paradigm is based on the individual as opposed to a community. This may be appropriate in individual consultations, but occupational physicians (OPs) also look after the health of communities of workers, so having *only* an individual focus for OH ethical guidance may be a further cause of this ethical confusion. This paper will explore whether adopting, or learning from, the ethical approaches used in public health (PH) could help in reducing the ethical confusion in OH practice.

Background

In the UK, the Faculty of Occupational Medicine (FOM) gives ethical guidance to OHPs and other occupational health professionals.[88] On the issue of confidentiality, it quotes the GMC guidance almost *verbatim*. GMC ethical guidance to all doctors is premised on a therapeutic doctor-patient relationship. This is understandable for most of medical practice. However, it has been argued that this ethical paradigm lacks coherence in some of the functions undertaken by UK OPs, for example, in writing independently commissioned reports for pension fund purposes. In that role, that paradigm would require an OP to be a fiduciary and independent at the same time,[89] which is clearly impossible.

If we are to look for an alternative ethical paradigm, could PH ethics be the answer? There is increasing overlap in the interests covered by PH and OH, such as health promotion programmes and environmental health. In OH we serve communities of

[83] Stern AF and Sperber S. Occupational physicians' perceptions and impact of 2009 GMC consent guidelines. *Occup Med (Lond)* 2012; **62**:560–562.

[84] Tamin J. Describing occupational medicine practice to establish a basis for ethical guidance. *Occup Med (Lond)* 2013; **63**:170–171.

[85] GMC. *Confidentiality: Supplementary guidance*. London 2009.

[86] Tamin J. Is the GMC guidance on confidentiality compatible with English law? *Occup Med (Lond)* 2015; **65**:266–267.

[87] Kloss D. Consent to occupational health reports. *Occup Med (Lond)* 2015; **65**:700–703.

[88] Faculty of Occupational Medicine, *Ethics Guidance for Occupational Health Practice*, 7th edition, Royal College of Physicians, London, December 2012.

[89] Tamin J. Models of occupational medicine practice: an approach to understanding moral conflict in "dual obligation" doctors. *Medicine, Health Care and Philosophy*, 2013; **16**:3, 499–506.

workers as well as the individual worker, whereas PH focuses mainly on community benefits. There may therefore be similarities as well as differences in the way ethical justifications are, or should be, deployed in OH and PH practice.

On the other hand, it could be said that *all* doctors have responsibilities to society, or other parties, as well as their patients. This will be discussed in the next section.

Dual Obligation Doctors

Although all doctors have at least some responsibilities to society, Gillon (1985) points out that: "despite this acceptance (of obligations to society) doctors often talk and think as if they believe that they invariably give absolute moral priority to their patients over the moral demands of society".[90] The GMC reinforce this message to doctors: "you must make the care of your patient your first concern" (GMC 2013).[91]

However, this may not be the case for OPs in practice, at least, not to the same extent. OPs have "dual obligations". The GMC state that "dual obligations arise when a doctor works for or is contracted (such as) by a patient's employer, an insurance company, an agency assessing a claimant's entitlement to benefits, the armed forces".[92] Similarly, the British Medical Association (BMA) describes these as "situations where doctors have clear obligations to a third party that can be in tension to the obligation to the patient".[93]

The obligations towards the individual patient versus society could be viewed as a continuum, where a treating doctor owes maximal obligation to his patient, whereas a PH doctor has maximal obligation to society. For OPs, their "dual" obligations would lie somewhere in between these two extremes.

This is illustrated by the following (Table C.1).

However, if we accept that OPs can be in different roles, ranging from a "quasi-therapeutic" to an "independent expert" one,[94] then the exact position for OPs along the x-axis would vary according to which role they were performing at the time. Thus at the right side of the x-axis, an OP in the "independent" role would have greater obligations to third parties than the "patient" (a term which is arguably a misnomer in OH practice), that is, apparently close to a PH doctor's position with regard to their obligations. It therefore seems reasonable to postulate some closeness between OH and PH ethics, at least at that end of the spectrum. What then, can we learn from PH ethics?

---

[90]Gillon R. 1985. *Philosophical medical ethics*, John Wiley & sons, Chichester, p. 158.

[91]GMC. 2013. *Good Medical Practice*, p. 4.

[92]GMC.2009. *Confidentiality: Supplementary guidance*, p. 24.

[93]BMA. 2012. *Medical Ethics Today: The BMA's Handbook of Ethics and Law*, 3rd edition, London, p. 649.

[94]See Tamin (2013), at ref (8) for a suggested account of OHP roles in different "models".

Table C.1 Obligations to society versus patient

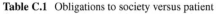

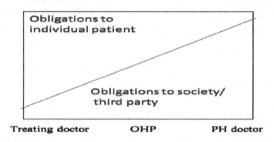

PH ethical approaches:

The Nuffield Council on Bioethics comments:

> The emphasis of public health policy on prevention rather than treatment of the sick, on the population as a whole rather than the individual, and the importance of collective effort, poses a particular set of ethical problems. In traditional bioethics, much emphasis is placed on the freedom of the individual, in terms of consent, treatment and information. Whilst these freedoms remain in ethical considerations of public health, they are woven into a complex fabric, in which many different players have roles and responsibilities.[95]

Some of this clearly resonates with OH practice. OH is also a preventive, rather than curative, specialty. On the other hand, it is concerned with the individual worker, *as well as* the collective. So, it may be reasonable to expect concerns about "individual freedom" to play a part in the ethical basis for consent and information in the OH context. However, when the collective interest is the more predominant (as with PH issues), how then does PH ethics address the ethical tensions? In order to explore this, examples that draw out issues in the PH arena, first around confidentiality and privacy, and secondly around consent, will next be discussed.

Practical examples:

1. *Health data sharing*

The Nuffield Council on Bioethics comments on the opportunities for linking and re-use of health data as follows:

> The continuing accumulation of data and the increasing power and availability of analytical tools mean that new opportunities arise, and will continue to arise, to extract value from data. There is a public interest in the responsible use of data to support the development of

---

[95]Nuffield Council on Bioethics. *Public health: ethical issues.* London: 2007, p. v.

knowledge and innovation through scientific research and to improve the well-being of all through improved health advice, treatment and care.[96]

It also points out that the increasing use of health data has become a "strategic focus"[97] in the NHS. However, this public interest in health improvements through the use of this data has to be balanced against our reasonable expectation of privacy of our health data. "Privacy is fundamentally important to individuals (and groups) in the establishment and maintenance of their identity, their relationships and their sense of personal well-being."[98] This tension between pursuing improvements in public health, and individual privacy, therefore needs to be addressed in data sharing programmes.

The best known type of the population research data initiatives is known as a "biobank", which involves different types of biological sample and data collection. In the UK, the UK Biobank is the largest, with more than 500,000 individuals recruited. The intention is to follow them for at least 25 years, through periodic collection of data, as well as through their GP and hospital records. From 2012, data from this biobank has been available to researchers worldwide for a modest fee. The UK Biobank Ethics and Governance Council oversees the research process, and is said to continually review the ethical framework in an open and reflective way. For this reason, it is felt that a "secure moral basis (is provided) for the proposed uses (of data) in most respects."[99]

However, the issue of data sharing is not uncontroversial. The relatively positive experience from the UK Biobank project was not replicated with the NHS England "care.data" programme. This programme has been particularly focused on GP data, as well as widening the scope of data collected from hospital records. Although it is claimed that this would lead to better care,[100] the project had been widely criticised.[101] More recently, the Independent Information Governance Oversight Panel (IIGOP), chaired by Dame Fiona Caldicott, produced a report[102] which sought various assurances, including that that patients would be appropriately informed and given opt out choices, and as long as those conditions are satisfied, the pilot stage would take place in 6 "pathfinder" GP practices. There is reported evidence of broad

---

[96]Nuffield Council on Bioethics. *The collection, linking and use of data in biomedical research and health care: ethical issues.* London: 2015, p. 23.

[97]At p. 22.

[98]Nuffield Council on Bioethics (2015), p. xv.

[99]Nuffield Council on Bioethics (2015), p. 136, para 7.21.

[100]http://www.nhs.uk/NHSEngland/thenhs/records/healthrecords/Documents/better-information-means-better-care.pdf, and O'Dowd A. Medical Data: Does patient privacy trump access for research? *BMJ*, 2013, **347**, 20–21.

[101]See for example http://www.dailymail.co.uk/news/article-2567980/Sharing-medical-files-harms-trust-says-BMA-Senior-doctors-warn-using-data-cause-irreversible-damage.html and Sterckx S, Rakic V, Cockbain J and Borry P. 2015. "You hoped we would sleep walk into accepting the collection of our data": controversies surrounding the UK care.data scheme and their wider relevance for biomedical research, *Medicine, Health Care and Philosophy.* https://doi.org/10.1007/s11019-015-9661-6.

[102]IIGOP. *Information—to share or not to share. 2014 Annual Report*, December 2014.

public support for their health data to be used for secondary purposes, including health service improvement or research, but "this support is said to fall away to a significant extent where they are not asked, or where the research involves private companies operating for profit."[103]

Although the Nuffield Council report proposes no easy solutions, it stresses the importance of "*participation* of those with morally relevant interests",[104] with a complementary "principle of *accounting for decisions*",[105] and recognises the fluidity of the social, scientific and political settings within which this balanced (that is, balancing privacy and public interests) oversight of privacy protection would operate. Crucially, such an approach is underpinned by complete *transparency* at each step of the development of privacy norms for any data initiatives.[106] The practical precepts for such initiatives include the continued involvement of stakeholders to reflect on and determine the morally important issues, values and interests, as well as the continuing review and governance of these initiatives.

It has been argued that such transparency is lacking in the current medical confidentiality paradigm,[107] so this may be an important lesson one could learn from PH ethics. This will be reviewed further in the discussion section, but first, the concept of consent will be explored, using the context of vaccination programmes.

2. *Vaccination programmes*

It has been said that "the ethical principle that underlies the doctrine of consent is that of patient autonomy".[108] In the context of vaccinations, and other therapeutic interventions, I agree with this assertion. However, in the context of information disclosed in an OH report, it is *privacy* rather than *autonomy*[109] that is the primary interest to be protected. I therefore suggest the concept of "permission to disclose" would be more appropriate in the situation of disclosing an OH report, rather than that of "informed consent". This issue does not concern us here, as we are interested in the concepts of informed consent and autonomy in vaccination programmes, and the difference between the two types of consent is only mentioned for clarification.

Returning to our interest in consent and autonomy, these clearly have primacy when our concern is with the individual, and an intervention is being considered. As the Nuffield Council (2007) points out, the "stress on the importance of individual autonomy implies that the concept of consent plays a key role".[110] One should note however, that it has been argued that simply choosing our "first order desires"[111]

---

[103] Nuffield Council on Bioethics (2015), p. 90, para 5.18.

[104] At p. 155, para 8.10.

[105] At p. 155, para 8.10.

[106] pp. 156–157.

[107] Tamin J. 2015. What are "patient secrets" in occupational medicine? Privacy and confidentiality in "dual obligation doctor" situations, *Medical Law International*, 15(1), pp. 19–48, at 43.

[108] Kloss (2015), at ref (6).

[109] Tamin J. Can informed consent apply to information disclosure? Moral and practical implications, *Clinical Ethics*, March 2014, 9, 1, 1–9.

[110] At p. 18.

[111] Dworkin G. *The theory and practice of autonomy*, Cambridge University Press, 1988, p. 15.

does not necessarily express our autonomy, and in order for us to be truly self-determining, we must opt for autonomy that is reflective and "principled".[112] The Nuffield Council also suggests that an ethical framework for public health needs to include values which emphasise the benefits to *all* members of society. Such an approach is often described as "solidarity" or "community" (the latter is the Nuffield Council's preferred term, although I prefer solidarity). This value is central in "the limitation on individual consent when it obstructs important general benefits".[113]

Vaccination can be of benefit to the vaccinated individual, and, if sufficient members of their community are vaccinated, that community also benefits through herd immunity. The ethical question that arises is whether the benefit to a community of having sufficient numbers of its members vaccinated to produce such herd immunity (assuming that a purely voluntary system does not recruit the required numbers), would ever be a justification for overriding individual consent. That is, whether it could be ever be morally justifiable to apply coercion or compulsion in order to achieve this wider benefit to society.

Before we can address this question, we would first need more information about the benefit of that vaccination programme to society, and any possible harm to the individual from being vaccinated. We would need to know how serious the infection itself was, whether prevention of transmission could be achieved in other ways, how effective the vaccine was, and the nature and severity of side-effects of the vaccine. One would therefore expect the answer to our ethical question to be different for different vaccines. Some vaccination programmes are carried out in an OH setting, for example influenza vaccination of healthcare workers (HCWs) to prevent nosocomial transmission. A recent in-depth review of such a programme concludes that "while vaccination of HCWs is necessary, on its own it may not be sufficient to prevent nosocomial influenza infection, and a multidimensional approach is clearly required."[114] The authors advocate that this approach should be a risk management one, to include a review of the hierarchy of controls in place to prevent nosocomial influenza transmission. This illustrates the need for any evaluation (of whether a vaccination programme should be voluntary or mandatory) to be done in its actual context, with all relevant factors taken into consideration.

So, could vaccination ever be made compulsory? Well, currently no truly compulsory vaccination programme exists. However, there are several examples of "quasi-mandatory" programmes, where those who are not vaccinated cannot access some benefit, such as access to education (for example, in France, Spain and the USA).[115] It could be argued that penalising children by denying them access to education is

---

[112]O'Neill O. *Autonomy and Trust in Bioethics, The Gifford Lectures 2001*, Cambridge University Press, 2002, p. 73–95.

[113]At p. 23.

[114]O'Reilly F, Dolan GP, Nguyen-Van-Tam J, Noone P. Practical prevention of nosocomial influenza transmission, 'a hierarchical control' issue. *Occup Med (Lond)* 2015; **65**; 696–700.

[115]Nuffield Council on Bioethics (2007), at p. 58.

itself morally repugnant,[116] so a balance needs to be struck between the benefits resulting from vaccination, and the harms arising from a quasi-mandatory approach, particularly from the sanctions that are used.

Most commentators first clarify that voluntariness is the preferable approach. However, if the numbers who volunteer to be vaccinated are not sufficient to produce herd immunity, and the infection is sufficiently serious, then these commentators contend that it is morally justifiable to consider more coercive approaches. Although direct compulsion would generally be regarded as "an action of last resort",[117] it has been argued that "on balance, a wholly voluntary vaccination programme may no longer be tenable, and reflection is needed about whether coercion may offer the way forward".[118] As for the Nuffield Council, it "identified two circumstances in which quasi-mandatory vaccination measures are more likely to be justified. First, for highly contagious and serious diseases, for example with characteristics similar to smallpox. Secondly, for disease eradication if the disease is serious and if eradication is within reach."[119]

Discussion

What lessons can we learn from these examples from PH ethics?

Confidentiality is hugely important in OM practice, as it is in the rest of medicine. However, confidentiality is not absolute, and breaches are allowed by the GMC and FOM, for example, if others could be harmed. In the language of *principlism*, these breaches would be justified on the basis of non-maleficence.[120] However, some commentators[121] contend that the fact that breaches are allowed at all equates to a lack of transparency in this version of confidentiality, and may lead to public *mistrust*, instead of the trust it is meant to engender.

In addition, it may seem ironic that, while the GMC places exacting controls on the fitness for work advice by an OP to an employer,[122] UK patients may have their much more sensitive health data (as contained in their GP records) communicated to a number of bodies and organisations. However, in the case of the UK Biobank, we see that with a transparent process and good information governance oversight,

---

[116] Glover-Thomas N and Holm S. *Compulsory vaccination*, in *Pioneering Healthcare Law*. (Stanton C, Devaney S et al., eds.). Routledge, Oxon. 2016, pp. 31–42, at p. 42.

[117] Dawson A. *Public health ethics: Key issues and concepts in policy and practice*. Cambridge University Press, Cambridge, 2011, at p. 151.

[118] Glover-Thomas N and Holm S (2016), at p. 42.

[119] Nuffield Council on Bioethics (2007), at p. 60.

[120] Beauchamp TL and Childress JF. *Principles of Biomedical Ethics*, 5th edition, 2001. Oxford University Press: New York, pp. 113–115.

[121] See for example: Kottow MH. Medical confidentiality: an intransigent and absolute obligation, *J Med Ethics*, 1986, 12, pp. 117–122; and Warwick SJ. A vote for no confidence, *J Med Ethics*, 1989, 15, pp. 183–5.

[122] GMC. *Confidentiality: Supplementary guidance*, London 2009, p 23.

there can be public trust in and support for, such data sharing. Whether a similar approach could work in the OM context is beyond the scope of this paper, but it has been considered elsewhere previously.[123]

On the issue of confidentiality, the main lesson I wish to draw out from the PH example of data sharing is that the ethical interest that confidentiality may need to be balanced against is not only non-maleficence, but could also be *beneficence,* which is said to refer to "an action done to benefit others".[124] The action of sharing health data is done with the intention of developing knowledge through research in order "to improve the well-being of all through improved health advice, treatment and care".[125] Maybe we already do apply the principle of beneficence to some extent in OM, for example when we disclose anonymised health surveillance data to employers as part of health surveillance programmes.[126] This information is shared with employers to help them protect their workforce. However, in the OM context, the need to share information to benefit a community is not made as explicit as the PH justification for health data sharing. The latter justification may therefore serve as a useful reminder to those of us practising OM that respect for privacy needs to be balanced not only against instances of non-maleficence, but also where a consideration of beneficence may be relevant.

The second example, that of vaccination programmes, is a situation where "informed consent" is the appropriate consideration, rather the concept of "permission to disclose" which is preferable in disclosing a report. The fact that "informed consent" originates from the Nuremberg trials for the Nazi horrors explains the importance we place on voluntariness. From the 1970's, autonomy has become the main justification for consent. It is therefore understandable that we recoil somewhat at the thought of any form of coercion. However, the PH ethics example of vaccination raises our awareness of the need to balance the needs of the community, and that *solidarity* is also a value that should be taken into account in these circumstances.

I am not suggesting that individual OPs should breach confidence, or override autonomy and consent. Instead, I would urge the rule makers and policy makers to have a more balanced view of these interests in the development of future OM ethics guidance, as a paradigm based only the individual can produce too narrow a view of the relevant ethical interests.

Conclusion

One cannot simply import the ethical approaches used in PH into OM practice. That would be just as inappropriate as transposing the whole ethical paradigm of therapeutic medicine onto OM and expect this to work seamlessly. Yet, this is the

---

[123]Tamin J (2015), pp. 45–47.
[124]Beauchamp and Childress (2001), p. 166.
[125]Nuffield Council on Bioethics (2015), p. 23.
[126]FOM (2012), p. 30.

current GMC and FOM approach to OM ethics. As we serve communities as well as individual workers in OM, we should be at least cognisant of the values of solidarity and benefit to a community, and balance these against our traditional ethical value of individual autonomy.

Appendix D
Ethics Reflection & Audit Tool in Occupational Health (ERATOH)

Ethics Reflection & Audit Tool in Occupational Health (ERATOH)

Type of OH Professional-worker relationship: *Quasi-therapeutic? Independent expert?*

Reference:

Date:

1. Ethical considerations	2. Worker	3. Area of Practice or Issues	4. Employer	5. Others
A. Dual obligations of OH Professional *N.B. Trust*	• Need for further evidence for diagnosis? • Uncertainty of diagnosis?	Diagnosis/problem	• Questions asked? • Organisational values	(i) (ii) (iii)
B. Autonomy Duty-based: legal, ethical, standards? Protection of worker health	• Consent to process? • Understanding? • Acceptance?	Work capacity	• H&S issues? • Adjustments?	• H&S issues?
C. Privacy Confidentiality *Dual obligations* Protection of worker health	• Advice • Permission to disclose?	Communication	• Report • Permission to disclose?	
D. Non-maleficence/Beneficence/Justice/Fairness *Are ethical demands in conflict?*	• Duty to worker?	Concerns/ Conflicts/ Consequences	• Duty to employer? • Conflicts of interest?	• Impact on family? • Duty to others?• Community? (think of solidarity)
E. Summary/self-reflection *What have I learnt?* *Would I do anything differently in future?*	Justifications for preferred ethical outcome *Balancing ethical tensions?*			

Guidance notes:

1. Select cases where you feel uneasy about the possible *ethical* issues
2. Do not include worker/employer etc. identifiable information
3. Concentrate on the **ethical** aspects of the case, rather than the clinical/technical aspects
4. Highlight the ethical areas/considerations that you feel are relevant
5. Add brief comments, e.g. as comment boxes, but feel free to adapt to suit your needs/preferences
6. Summarise main issues for reflection
7. If possible, discuss your reflections with peers, e.g. in your audit group.

Appendix E
An Example Using the Ethics Reflection & Audit Tool in Occupational Medicine (ERATOM)

Ethics Reflection & Audit Tool in Occupational Medicine (ERATOM)
Type of OP-worker relationship: *Quasi-therapeutic?*
Independent expert? (e.g. for some Pension schemes)

Reference: EG

Date: 7 July 2016

© Springer Nature Switzerland AG 2020
J. Tamin, *Occupational Health Ethics*,
https://doi.org/10.1007/978-3-030-47283-2

Ethical considerations	Worker 45 year old male supervisor	Area	Employer chemical manufacturer	Others
				1. neighbouring community 2. 3.
Dual obligations of OP Trust	• Need for further evidence for diagnosis? • Uncertainty of diagnosis? Also poorly controlled DM type 2, marked postural bp drop noted, has felt dizzy on exertion 2 yrs	Diagnosis/problem Fall from ladder at work 2 days before, having private physio paid by employer, for soft tissue injuries	• Questions asked? Only re: FFW, not about cause of fall • Organisational values	
Autonomy Duty-based: legal, ethical, standards?	• Consent to process? Open and honest, consented to process• Understanding? Understood issues • Acceptance? yes	Work capacity note: usual duties supervisory, rarely physical	• H&S issues? Yes possibly • Adjustments?	• H&S issues? Yes possibly
Dual obligations Privacy Confidentiality	• Advice To see GP for DM control, refer to specialist for orthostatic hypotension • Permission to disclose? Yes	Communication	• Report advised fit for sedentary duties in a few days, restricted from physical work for longer term, to be reviewed in 4 weeks • Permission to disclose? Yes	
Non-maleficence/Beneficence/Justice/Fairness *Are ethical demands in conflict?*	• Duty to worker?	Concerns/ Conflicts/ Consequences worker concerned employer could stop paying for physio if underlying condition declared, and may be dismissed	• Duty to employer? Must be truthful, but employer did not ask about causation. Remaining H&S concern, but usual duties supervisory, where he would be safe • Conflicts of interest?	• Impact on family? • Duty to other workers? Remaining H&S concern, but usual duties supervisory, where he would be safe • Community? (think of solidarity)

(continued)

(continued)

Ethical considerations	Worker 45 year old male supervisor	Area	Employer chemical manufacturer	Others 1. neighbouring community 2. 3.
Summary/Self-reflection *What have I learnt?* *Would I do anything differently?*		Justifications for preferred ethical outcome/Resolution? I decided not to disclose underlying condition could have contributed to fall. Is this justified? Could be residual H&S risk, mitigated by restricting him from work that might trigger symptoms. However, if postural hypotension cannot be improved, and employer insists that some element of physical work required in his role after the 4 weeks, the ethical tensions will re-surface. Also, other OPs may take another line, so ethical issues worth discussion in group.		

Guidance notes:

8.   Select cases where you feel uneasy about the possible *ethical i*ssues
9.   Do not include worker/employer etc. identifiable information
10. Concentrate on the **ethical** aspects of the case, rather than the clinical/technical aspects
11. Highlight the ethical areas/considerations that you feel are relevant
12. Add brief comments, e.g. as comment boxes, but feel free to adapt to suit your needs/preferences
13. Summarise main issues for reflection
14. If possible, discuss your reflections with peers, e.g. in your audit group.

Notes

Notes to Prologue

1. International Commission on Occupational Health (ICOH), International Code of Ethics for Occupational Health Professionals, 3rd edition, 2014, at p. 16: "The duties of occupational health professionals include protecting the life and the health of the worker, **respecting human dignity** and promoting the highest ethical principles in occupational health policies and programmes." (my emphasis).

Notes to Chap. 1

Introduction

1. In Beauchamp TL and Childress JF. Principles of Biomedical Ethics. 2013. Cambridge University Press, 7th edition, "ethics" is defined thus: "*Ethics* is a generic term covering several different ways of understanding and examining the moral life." (p. 1). *Morality* "refers to norms about right and wrong human conduct that are so widely shared that they form a stable social compact." (pp. 2–3). I will use the terms ethics and morality, and ethical and moral, interchangeably throughout the book.
2. International Commission on Occupational Health (ICOH). International Code of Ethics for Occupational Health Professionals. 3rd edition, 2014, at p. 11:

   1. The aim of occupational health practice is to protect and promote workers' health, to sustain and improve their working capacity and ability, to contribute to the establishment and maintenance of a safe and healthy working environment for all, as well as to promote the adaptation of work to the capabilities of workers, taking into account their state of health.

© Springer Nature Switzerland AG 2020
J. Tamin, *Occupational Health Ethics*,
https://doi.org/10.1007/978-3-030-47283-2

2. The field of occupational health is broad and covers the prevention of all impairments arising out of employment, work injuries and work-related disorders, including occupational diseases and all aspects relating to the interactions between work and health. Occupational health professionals should be involved, whenever possible, in the design and choice of health and safety equipment, appropriate methods and procedures and safe work practices and they should encourage workers' participation in this field as well as feedback from experience.

Integrity

3. ICOH, International Code of Ethics for Occupational Health Professionals, 3rd edition, 2014. *Integrity* is highlighted in: "**Integrity in professional conduct**, impartiality and the protection of the confidentiality of health data and of the privacy of workers are part of these duties." (p. 16, emphasis added).
4. For an example of other health care professionals having pressures to act in ways that could be contrary to a patient's best interest, consider the situation where the state offers financial incentives for family doctors if they achieve certain targets, such as to achieve a certain percentage rate for immunizations or cervical cancer screening of their practice populations. There could be good public health reasons for such incentives, and there may be benefit for the individual patient.
5. However, there may also be conflicts of interest, where a doctor needs to guard against breaching his professional integrity. For further comment on this, see Bartlett P. Doctors as fiduciaries: Equitable regulation of the doctor-patient relationship. Medical Law Review. 1997, 5, pp. 193–224, at p. 216.

Why OH ethics?

6. Faculty of Occupational Medicine, Guidance on ethics for occupational physicians, 6th edition, London: Faculty of Occupational Medicine of the Royal College of Physicians, May 2006. This is an earlier edition on the Faculty of Occupational Medicine's Ethics Guidance, from which I quote Dr. David Snashall's comments in the main text.
7. Martimo KP, Antti-Poika M, Leinof T and Rossit K. Ethical issues among Finnish occupational physicians and nurses. Occupational Medicine. 1998, 48, pp. 375–380. Their study of 200 OH physicians and nurses reported that 97% of them had experienced ethical issues in their OH practice.
8. Iavicoli S, Valenti A, Gagliardi D, Rantanen J. Ethics and Occupational Health in the Contemporary World of Work. Int. J. Environ. Res. Public Health. 2018, 15, 1713; https://doi.org/10.3390/ijerph15081713. The authors cite one of several contributors to the increase in OH ethical dilemmas as being "the development of a multidisciplinary approach in occupational health (i.e., technical, medical, social and legal), which implies the involvement of other specialists who belong to various professions in occupational health services." A corollary to this observation, I believe, must be that **all** OH professionals should follow the same ethical code, such as the ICOH International Code of Ethics (2014).

Codes of ethics

9. Westerholm P. Codes of ethics—Are they important? Ethical dilemmas and challenges in occupational health. CME Nov/Dec 2009 Vol. 27 No. 11, pp. 492–494. "The key issue in discussing ethical codes is the extent to which they can be utilised to enhance moral awareness and thereby earn the trust of clients and the public." (p. 493); and "Ethical codes should be seen as powerful bearers of the traditional value sets of occupational health professionals." (p. 494). I could not agree more with the author's comments.

10. Westerholm P. Professional Ethics in Occupational Health- Western European Perspectives. Industrial Health, 2007, 45, pp. 19–25. "There is certainly a need for such norms even if one is well advised to be aware of the limitations of such guidelines. It is commonly accepted that it is not possible to draft rules providing detailed guidance in the many differing situations dealt with by occupational health professionals at work." (p. 23); and "Codes are commonly aspirational and well intentioned, but most often not enforceable. They vary significantly in clarity, depth, emphasis, strength and relevance. The reader commonly finds no guidance in them for resolving of ethical dilemmas. (p. 24). I believe these observations to be helpful and uncontroversial.

11. Westerholm P, Nilstun T, Ovretveit J (Eds.). Practical ethics in occupational health. Radcliffe Medical Press. 2004. Chapter 24, entitled "Professional codes of ethics": "codes may be helpful and even necessary as a moral compass-providing guidance and important reminders". (p. 328). Once again, I cite this in agreement.

12. See also Tamin J. Ethics guidance for occupational health practice: a commentary. Clinical Ethics. 2014, 9 (2–3), pp. 61–62. In this commentary on a previous iteration of the UK guidance, I make the point that it would be helpful for practitioners to understand the basis for advice given in the guidance in certain situations (I use the example of information from OH to the worker's GP). This would allow OH practitioners to better understand how to apply the guidance when faced with their own ethical problems.

13. Iavicoli et al. (2018): "Public and private institutions as well as organisations employing OHPs should adopt a programme of organisational ethics aligned with the ethical principles of ICOH Code (art. 19). The importance of the ICOH Code is reflected by the fact that national legislations (Argentina and Italy), international organizations (ILO, CIOMS, WHO), and other codes of ethics, post-graduate courses or treatises contain references to the subject. As far as the Italian national legal framework is concerned, pursuant to art. 39, c. 1 of Legislative Decree 81/08, "the activity of occupational physician is executed under the principles of occupational health and ICOH Code of Ethics." (p. 8). I agree with the authors that this paragraph demonstrates the importance and influence of the ICOH Code.

Scope of this book

14. Although this book does not address the topic of research in OH, note the guidance from ICOH (2014): "Occupational health professionals involved in

research must design and carry out their activities on a sound scientific basis with full professional independence and follow the ethical principles relevant to health and medical research work. These include social and scientific value, scientific validity, fair subject selection, favourable risk benefit ratio, informed consent, respect for potential and enrolled subjects, review of protocols and potential conflicts of interest by an independent and competent ethics committee and protection of confidential data. The occupational health professionals have a duty to make their research results publicly available. They are accountable for the accuracy of their reports." (p. 22, para. 15).

15. For those who are interested in reading about the ethics of OH research, I would recommend Coggon D. Chapter 18: Occupational health research (pp. 241–251) in Westerholm P, Nilstun T, Ovretveit J (Eds.). Practical ethics in occupational health. Radcliffe Medical Press. 2004.

Moral theories and approaches

16. Beauchamp TL and Childress JF. Principles of Biomedical Ethics. 2013. Cambridge University Press, 7th edition. See especially the section on "Moral principles", pp. 101–340. The 1st edition was published in 1979.

17. Stanley JM, The Appleton Consensus: suggested international guidelines for decisions to forego medical treatment. Journal of Medical Ethics. 1989, 15, pp. 129–136.

18. Singer P. (Ed.) A companion to ethics.1993, Blackwell. For those who are interested in the deontology theories, see O'Neil O. Kantian ethics (chapter 14) and Davis NA. Contemporary deontology (chapter 17).

19. United Nations. 1948. Universal Declaration of Human Rights. Accessed at http://www.un.org/en/universal-declaration-human-rights/. I have selected some Articles that are particularly interesting to us: "Article 3: Everyone has the right to life, liberty and security of person."; "Article 12: No one shall be subjected to arbitrary interference with his privacy, family, home or correspondence, nor to attacks upon his honour and reputation. Everyone has the right to the protection of the law against such interference or attacks."; and especially the Article that pertains to work and working conditions, "Article 23: 1. Everyone has the right to work, to free choice of employment, to just and favourable conditions of work and to protection against unemployment. 2. Everyone, without any discrimination, has the right to equal pay for equal work. 3. Everyone who works has the right to just and favourable remuneration ensuring for himself and his family an existence worthy of human dignity, and supplemented, if necessary, by other means of social protection."

20. Westerholm P provides a comprehensive look at "Work and human rights" in chapter 1 of Westerholm P, Nilstun T, Ovretveit J (Eds.). Practical ethics in occupational health. Radcliffe Medical Press. 2004, pp. 5–7.

21. See also Dworkin R. Taking rights seriously. Bloomsbury Academic: 2013. The author provides a staunch defence of a rights-based approach: "Individual rights are political trumps held by individuals." (p. 6).

22. For an overview of consequentialist theories, see Pettit P. Consequentialism, chapter 9, pp. 230–240, in Singer P. (Ed.) A companion to ethics. 1993, Blackwell.
23. For background reading on utilitarianism, see Hare RM. A Utilitarian Approach, chapter 9, pp. 85–90, in Kuhse H and Singer P (Eds.). A Companion to Bioethics. 2012. Wiley-Blackwell, 2nd edition.

Notes to Chap. 2

The doctor-patient relationship and dual obligations in Occupational Health
The doctor-patient relationship

1. See O'Neill O. A Question of Trust. 2002, Cambridge University Press. She describes the doctor-patient relationship as "a paradigm of a relationship of trust...It is a professional relationship that is supposed to be disinterested, intimate and trusting" (at p. 17).
2. See Brazier M and Lobjoit M. Fiduciary relationship: An ethical approach and a legal concept? in Bennett R and Erin CA (Eds.). HIV and AIDS testing: Screening and confidentiality. 1999, Oxford University Press, pp. 179–199. For example, they remind us that "Patients trust doctors, **nurses and other health professionals** with intimate details of their lives which they may conceal even from their families." (at p. 187). I have highlighted "nurses and other health professionals" in bold, to indicate that this trust does not just apply to *doctors*, but also to *other* healthcare professionals.
3. See also Beauchamp TL and Childress JF. Principles of Biomedical Ethics. 2013. Cambridge University Press, 7th edition: "The virtues of honesty, truthfulness and candor are among deservedly praised character traits of health professionals and researchers." (at p. 302). Candor, honesty and truthfulness are certainly character traits that make healthcare professionals trust*worthy*, so these are the traits that we should maintain and develop in our OH practice.
4. I recognize that there is not just one type of "doctor-patient relationship". However, I have not mentioned this in the main text as I believe that patient trust remains important in all the different models of the relationship. For comment on some of the models, see Brody H. The Physician-Patient Relationship: Models and Criticisms. Theoretical Medicine 8. 1987, D. Reidel Publishing Company, pp. 205–220.
5. O'Neill (2002) says the following: "I might trust my GP (general practitioner, also known as family practitioner) to diagnose and prescribe for a sore throat, but not for a heart attack", and also "nurses and GPs are more trusted than hospital consultants" (at pp. 9–10).
6. See for example, Plomp HN and Ballast N. Trust and vulnerability in doctor-patient relations in occupational health. Occupational Medicine. 2010, 60,

pp. 261–269. This was a study carried out in the Netherlands. The authors suggest that "Where physician's independence, agency or expertise is questioned, distrust is harder to overcome." They also found that workers who were more "vulnerable" (for example, more seriously ill) or had work-related concerns were more likely to trust occupational physicians, but the responses were not uniform.

7. See also Plomp HN. Workers' attitude toward the occupational physician. Journal of Occupational Medicine. 1992, 34, 9, pp. 893–901.

In this study, again carried out in the Netherlands over 25 years ago (so some degree of distrust in OH is not new), the author found that "A negative evaluation of the OHS is mainly because of unclarity and uncertainty as to how the occupational physician combines his/her responsibility toward individual workers with his/her responsibility toward the company.", at p. 893.

8. Similarly, in a small survey in the UK, one third of workers thought the occupational physician would "favor the manager" after their OH consultation; (in Stilz R and Madan I. Worker expectations of occupational health consultations. Occupational Medicine. 2014, 64, pp. 177–180, in Table 1, at p. 178.) The authors point out that this was a survey of health care workers with an in-house service, so their results may not be applicable to other workers. However, once again, there is unfortunately some reported mistrust of OH services.

Dual obligations

9. See Sieghart P. Professional ethics- for whose benefit? Journal of Medical Ethics. 1982, pp. 25–32. Sieghart described the tension that arises from "trying to satisfy the worker and the employer at the same time", as "two-master ethics". The occupational physician had to grapple with the moral problems presented to him "when he finds that he owes different obligations, at the same time and in the same circumstances, to different people with conflicting interests". This remains an apt description of what is nowadays described as "dual obligations".

10. "Dual obligation doctors" are described for example in General Medical Council. Confidentiality: Disclosing information for employment, insurance and similar purposes. 2017. p. 2, para. 4, as follows: "Usually, dual obligations arise when a doctor works for, is contracted by, or otherwise provides services to: a patient's employer (as an occupational health doctor; an insurance company; an agency assessing a claimant's entitlement to benefits; the police (as a police surgeon); the armed forces; the prison service; a sports team or association".

Duty to workers

11. ICOH International Code of Ethics for Occupational Health Professionals (2014): "The aim of occupational health practice is to protect and promote workers' health, to sustain and improve their working capacity and ability, to contribute to the establishment and maintenance of a safe and healthy working environment for all, as well as to promote the adaptation of work to the capabilities of workers, taking into account their state of health." (at p. 11); and: "Occupational health professionals must always act, as a matter of prime

concern, in the interest of the health and safety of the workers." (at p. 23, para. 16).

12. For a description of, and discussion and balancing of, the four principles, see Beauchamp TL and Childress JF. Principles of biomedical ethics, 7th edition. 2013, Oxford University Press, pp. 13–25.

Duty to the employer

13. ICOH (2014): "The occupational health professionals must provide **competent and honest advice to the employers on fulfilling their responsibility in the field of occupational safety and health** as well as to the workers on the protection and promotion of their health in relation to work." (p. 17, emphasis added).

14. ICOH (2014): "Occupational health professionals must request that a clause on ethics be incorporated in their contract of employment. This clause on ethics should include, in particular, their right to apply professional standards, guidelines and codes of ethics. Occupational health professionals must not accept conditions of occupational health practice which do not allow for their functions according to the desired professional standards and principles of ethics." (p. 24).

15. Laurie GT, Harmon SHE and Porter G. Mason and McCall Smith's Law and Medical Ethics. 2016, 10th edition. Oxford University Press, at p. 205: "It must now be stated explicitly before carrying out a pre-employment medical examination, or a fitness to work, that the results of that examination may be communicated to the employer and the written consent of the examinee should be obtained in the light of that information. Likewise, in the case of examinations carried out for insurance purposes, the doctor must obtain the positive agreement of the patient to waive the normal obligations of confidentiality within a 'need to know' formula. In the absence of such agreement, it is unlikely that the doctor engaged in industrial or insurance medicine could justify, on either ethical or legal grounds, a breach of a patient's confidence on the grounds that he, the doctor, owed a duty as an employee to his employer." As I mention in the main text, I fully agree with this view. Although the authors refer to "doctor" here, I believe that this applies to all other OH professionals as well.

16. ICOH (2014): "Occupational health professionals are obliged not to reveal industrial or commercial secrets of which they become aware in the exercise of their activities. However, they must not withhold information which is necessary to protect the safety and health of workers or of the community." (p. 19).

17. For an insightful description and analysis of whistleblowing in OH practice, see the chapter "Whistleblowing" by Nilstun T. and Westerholm P., in Westerholm P, Nilstun T, Ovretveit J (Eds.). Practical ethics in occupational health. Radcliffe Medical Press. 2004, pp. 283–290.

Duty to other parties

18. Please note that throughout this book, whenever terms such as he or she, his or hers etc., are used, these are intended to be gender neutral. They will most often

be used merely for clarification, to differentiate between two different actors and these terms could be interchanged.

19. Gillon R. Philosophical medical ethics. 1985. John Wiley & sons, Chichester: "despite this acceptance (of obligations to society) doctors often talk and think as if they believe that they invariably give absolute moral priority to their patients over the moral demands of society". However, it might be argued that doctors' attitudes have changed over the last 30 years. Nonetheless, I think that doctors and other healthcare professionals still make "the patient their first concern" (and rightly so), so other considerations become secondary.

A fiduciary relationship?

20. For comment on the power imbalance between doctors and patients, see Kennedy I. The fiduciary relationship and its application to doctors and patients, in Wrongs and Remedies in the twenty-first century, (Ed. Birks P), Oxford University Press. 1996, pp. 111–140: "The doctor-patient relationship has special, perhaps unique, features. Principal among these is the very significant disequilibrium of power between the two parties. The patient is uniquely vulnerable, being not only ignorant of the expertise constituted by the practice of medicine but also, in most cases, ill and anxious or anxious about possibly being ill. By contrast, the doctor has expert knowledge." (at p. 111).

21. For example, see Brazier M and Lobjoit M. Fiduciary Relationship: An Ethical Approach and a Legal Concept? in Bennett R and Erin CA (Eds), HIV and AIDS testing: Screening and Confidentiality. Oxford University Press. 1999, pp. 179–199. They propose (at p. 180) that a "therapeutic alliance" between doctors and patients would be "best represented by developing the concept of the fiduciary relationship between patient and professional". They suggest that recognizing the fiduciary nature of that relationship would have several benefits for healthcare:

  (i)   Partnership will be placed at the centre of the agenda between the parties to the relationship.
  (ii) Within a partnership the focus shifts from patients in general to that particular patient with whom partnership is forged.
  (iii) Recognition can be given to the fact that both partners have responsibilities as well as rights. Reciprocity of obligations can be given real meaning.
  (iv) Establishing the parameters of the partnership between individual patients and professionals allows society to make a better-informed and more reflective judgment on when, if at all, obligations derived from that partnership may be overridden by obligations owed to society.

I find their arguments for such a fiduciary relationship quite compelling, and this approach also addresses the issue of the healthcare professional's balancing her obligations to her patient with her obligations to society.

22. For legal comment, see *Norberg* v. *Wynrib* [1992] 2 S.C.R. 226, 1–102, where McLachlin J delivered her seminal analysis of the doctor as a fiduciary:

> The doctor-patient relationship can be conceptualized as a creature of contract or tort but its most fundamental characteristic, rooted in the trust inherent in the relationship, is its fiduciary nature. (p. 6).

She then went on to explain her reasons for affirming the fiduciary nature of this relationship (p. 7):

> A fiduciary relationship is marked by the following characteristics:
>
> (1) the fiduciary has scope for the exercise of some discretion or power; (2) the fiduciary can unilaterally exercise that power or discretion so as to affect the beneficiary's legal or practical interests; and (3) the beneficiary is peculiarly vulnerable or at the mercy of the fiduciary holding the discretion or power. A physician owes his or her patient the classic duties associated with a fiduciary relationship—"loyalty, good faith, and avoidance of conflict of duty and self-interest".
>
> I think it is readily apparent that the doctor-patient relationship shares the peculiar hallmark of the fiduciary relationship—trust, the trust of a person with inferior power that another person who has assumed superior power and responsibility will exercise that power for his or her good and only for his or her good and in his or her best interests. Recognizing the fiduciary nature of the doctor-patient relationship provides the law with an analytic model by which physicians can be held to the high standards of dealing with their patients which the trust accorded them requires.

It is to be noted however that the doctor-patient relationship is recognised as being a fiduciary one *in law* in some parts of the world, such Canada, Australia and the United States, but not others, such as the United Kingdom.

23. See Bartlett P. Doctors as fiduciaries: Equitable regulation of the doctor-patient relationship. Medical Law Review, 5. 1997, pp. 193–224. He suggests that in terms of the scope of fiduciary duties, there are "four central principles" which he considers to be core values:

    i.   Fiduciaries must avoid conflicts of interest, or indeed even possible conflicts of interest, with the vulnerable party;
    ii. Fiduciaries must not profit from their position without prior disclosure to and authorisation from the vulnerable party;
    iii. The fiduciary owes a duty of undivided loyalty to the vulnerable party;
    iv. The fiduciary owes a duty of confidentiality to the vulnerable party. (at p. 198).

Independence

24. ICOH (2012): "Occupational professionals are experts who must enjoy **full professional independence** in the execution of their functions." (p. 16), and "Occupational health professionals must seek and maintain **full professional independence** and observe the rules of confidentiality in the execution of their functions. Occupational health professionals must under no circumstances allow their judgement and statements to be influenced by any conflict of interest, in particular when advising the employer, the workers or their representatives in the undertaking on occupational hazards and situations which present evidence of danger to health or safety. Such conflicts may distort the integrity of the

occupational health professionals who must ensure that the harm does not accrue with respect to workers' health and public health as a result of conflicts." (p. 23, para. 17). Emphases added.

25. See for example, the French Code de Déontologie Médicale (Avril 2017). Article 5—indépendance professionnelle. It is stressed that a doctor must remain professionally independent in all circumstances. (Le médecin ne peut aliéner son indépendance professionnelle sous quelque forme que ce soit).

26. In the UK, the term "independent" is used, for example, in the title "Independent Registered Medical Practitioner" (IRMP) in the Local Government Pension Scheme (Benefits, Membership and Contributions) Regulations 2014. The IRMP signs the certificate including the following statement: "I have not previously advised, or given an opinion on, or otherwise been involved in this case, nor am I acting or have ever acted as the representative of the member, the scheme employer or any other party in relation to it". Similar terminology and approach is used in some other UK public sector pension schemes, such as "IQMP" (Independent Qualified Medical Practitioner) for the Firefighters' Pension Scheme 2015.

OH Professional roles

27. For a fuller elaboration of the OH professional roles (discussing the physician roles, but the same approach can be applied to other healthcare professionals), see Tamin J. Models of occupational medicine practice: an approach to understanding moral conflict in "dual obligation" doctors. Medicine, Healthcare and Philosophy. 2013, 16(3), pp. 499–506. https://doi.org/10.1007/s11019-012-9426-4. A copy is at Appendix 1. In this article, I also suggest a further role which I call "impartial", which would be between the "quasi-therapeutic" and "independent" ones. On further reflection, I think we could define several different roles between the ends of that spectrum of roles. I will not be exploring these further possible roles in this book.

28. For examples of coercion of OH professionals by workers, see Baron C and Poole J. Organizations and illness deception among employees, in Halligan PW, Bass C and Oakley DA (Eds.). Malingering and illness deception. Oxford University Press. 2003, p. 248: "In extreme cases, colleagues (OPs) have been described being threatened, complained about to their employers or reported to the General Medical Council by patients who were unhappy that their claim for financial benefit was not supported. We have also encountered patients who have asked for information to be removed from medical reports which did not support their claim for financial benefits".

29. See also, Ghani R. Complaints against healthcare workers. Occupational Health at Work. 2017. 14(2), pp. 13–18, for an account of coercion and attempts at suppressing unfavourable OH professionals' IHR reports by applicants (at p. 15).

Conclusion

30. Westerholm P. Professional Ethics in Occupational Health- Western European Perspectives. Industrial Health, 2007, 45, pp. 19–25: "One basic principle to keep uppermost in the minds of occupational health professionals dealing with multiple loyalties is transparency and unmistakable declaration of own role in agreements, contracts and commitments." (p. 23). I agree that **transparency** of our roles and dual obligations (or multiple loyalties) are key to gaining the trust of workers, employers and others.

31. I suggest that if we develop an ethical paradigm or framework for OH, it should be built on the recognition of our "dual obligations" and our primary duty to protect the health of workers (see chapter 9). I will emphasize this approach throughout the book. For an equivalent approach in Public Health Ethics (based on different normative factors which are relevant in Public Health), see Dawson A (Ed.). Public Health Ethics: Key concepts and issues in policy and practice. 2011. Cambridge University Press, pp. 12–18.

Notes to Chap. 3

Consent
Origins of consent

1. The origins of the concept of consent could arguably be traced further back than the Nuremberg trials. For example, Kant's second Categorical Imperative "not to treat the humanity in a person simply as a means to an end, but always at the same time as an end" (paraphrased), can be seen as expressing respect for persons. From this perspective, a person cannot consent to being used merely as a means to an end. See O'Neill O. "Kantian ethics" in Singer P. (Ed.) "A companion to ethics". 1993, Blackwell, pp. 178–179.

2. However, in terms of consent for medical research, the Nuremberg Code 1947 (https://history.nih.gov/research/downloads/nuremberg.pdf) provides the clearest and most authoritative statement of the need for consent in this context. As mentioned in the main text, the concept was later extended to include therapeutic interventions.

Autonomy

3. For a fuller account of definitions and conceptions of autonomy, see Dworkin G. The theory and practice of autonomy. 1988, Cambridge University Press, pp. 3–20.

4. See Manson NC and O'Neill O. Rethinking Informed Consent in Bioethics. 2007, Cambridge University Press, pp. 19–21, for their discussion on conceptions of autonomy, including those that reflect "mere choice" as opposed to "reasoned or reflective choice".

Trust and autonomy

5. For an illuminating discussion on the relationship between trust and autonomy, see Onora O'Neill's first chapter entitled "Gaining autonomy and losing trust?", in her book entitled "Autonomy and Trust in Bioethics". 2002, Cambridge University Press, at pp. 1–27.
6. See also Manson NC and O'Neill O. (2007): "A suspicion of trust is central to contemporary autonomy-based bioethics, and typically reflects fears that trust can be misplaced, and that the cost of trusting the untrustworthy can be high", at p. 158.
7. I have previously argued that autonomy points to greater *independence*, whereas trust points to greater *inter-dependence*, so are arguably inversely related. See Tamin J. Can informed consent apply to information disclosure? Moral and practical implications. Clinical Ethics. 2014, Vol. 9(1), pp. 1–9, at p. 3.

Relational autonomy

8. For an account of relational autonomy in the healthcare context, see Tauber AI. Patient autonomy and the ethics of responsibility. 2005, MIT Press, pp. 112–123.
9. If Albert does *not* change his mind after further reflection, even within this relation of trust, then Allison must respect his choice, and not disclose to the manager. Is this then a waste of Allison's time? I feel not. I believe that Albert's further reflection with Allison's help is still of value. He will have made a more considered decision and be more aware of the possible consequences. I would also suggest that OH advisers like Allison (many of whom I have had the privilege of working with) are a credit to the OH profession and raise the level of trust in OH generally.

Solidarity

10. Solidarity is a term and concept used in Public Health ethics. Other terms for solidarity are *community* and *fraternity*. See Nuffield Council on Bioethics. Public health: ethical issues. 2007. ISBN: 978-1-904384-17-5, p. 23. The Nuffield Council prefers the term community. I prefer solidarity, as it is the term more often used in Public Health ethics literature.
11. In an OH context, solidarity is mentioned in Westerholm P, Nilstun T, Ovretveit J (Eds.). Practical ethics in occupational health. Radcliffe Medical Press. 2004. See for example at p. 113, where it is used to explain the principle of justice, in the context of social security arrangements which are based on solidarity. I fully agree with their approach but I believe that other sources (such as codes of ethics) should also use solidarity more explicitly and more often in their OH ethical analyses.
12. A definition of solidarity is given in Prainsac B and Buyx A. Solidarity: reflections on an emerging concept in bioethics. 2011. A report commissioned by the Nuffield Council on Bioethics. ISBN: 978-1-904384-25-0, as follows: "solidarity signifies shared practices reflecting a collective commitment to carry 'costs' (financial, social, emotional, or otherwise) to assist others.", at p. 46.

13. Prainsac and Buyx (2011) in their preferred relational model, explain that auton- omy and solidarity can be co-exist equally in the following way: "because the individual is seen as emerging from the relations in which she is embedded, solidarity is at least of equal importance to individual rights and interests. None of the two, communal or individual interest, a priori weighs more heavily or overrules the other." (at p. 52).

What does this mean for consent?

14. See Kloss D. Occupational Health Law. 2010, 5th edition, Wiley-Blackwell, pp. 220–221, for a legal perspective. UK case law generally rejects paternalism, except where the risk to the worker from continued employment is very high. However, she also cites the US case of *Echazabal v. Chevron USA Inc.* (2002), where the Supreme Court upheld the employer in their decision not to employ an oil refinery worker with hepatitis C, as he was more susceptible to liver damage from chemical exposure, even though he was disabled under the Americans with Disabilities Act. This is a case where paternalism overruled autonomy.

Informed consent

15. See Beauchamp TL. Autonomy and consent, in Miller FG and Wertheimer A (Eds). The ethics of consent. Oxford University Press, 2010: 55–78, at p. 55: "In biomedical ethics the language of 'consent' has been framed entirely as '*informed* consent'".
16. There is similar emphasis in the legal context on the *information* given to the con- senting individual. For example, Beauchamp TL. Informed consent: Its history, meaning and present challenges. Cambridge Quarterly of Healthcare Ethics. 2011, 20, pp. 515–523, at p. 518: "in the United States…informed consent has often been treated as synonymous with this legal doctrine, which is centred **almost entirely on disclosure** and on liability for injury" (emphasis added).
17. ICOH (2014) states the following on informed consent and health surveillance (at p. 20):

> The surveillance must be carried out with the non-coerced informed consent of the workers. The potentially positive and negative consequences of participation in screening and health surveillance programmes should be discussed as part of the consent process.

Permission to disclose

18. In the article: Tamin J. Can informed consent apply to information disclosure? Moral and practical implications. Clinical Ethics. 2014, Vol 9(1), pp. 1–9, I argued that permission to disclose protected privacy *rather* than autonomy. On further reflection, I would now say that it protects privacy *as well as* autonomy.

Conflation of the term "consent"

19. I have previously described the case of a healthcare worker sustaining a needle- stick injury where the donor patient is thought to be HIV positive, in Tamin J (2014), at pp. 5–6.

Capacity

20. For a discussion of competence, see Beauchamp TL and Childress JF. Principles
    of biomedical ethics, 7th edition. 2013, Oxford University Press, pp. 114–120.
    "Standards of competence feature mental skills or capacities closely connected
    to attributes of autonomous persons, such as cognitive skills and independent
    judgment. In criminal law, civil law, and clinical medicine, standards for com-
    petence cluster around various abilities to comprehend and process information
    and to reason about the consequences of one's actions. In medical contexts,
    physicians usually consider a person competent if he or she can understand a
    procedure, deliberate with regard to its major risks and benefits, and make a
    decision in light of this deliberation." (at p. 117).
21. ICOH (2014) at p. 11, para. 3: "On the basis of the principle of equity, occupa-
    tional health professionals should assist workers in obtaining and maintaining
    employment notwithstanding their health deficiencies **or their handicap**." (my
    emphasis). I very much agree that OH professionals should assist in the employ-
    ment of those who might otherwise be disadvantaged through physical or mental
    health conditions. The issue of competence to give consent is one area where
    OH professionals can assist in ensuring fair and equitable treatment of those
    with severe mental health conditions.
22. For a discussion of consent and non-competence, see Manson and O'Neill
    (2007), pp. 192–194. In the context of treatment, they maintain that "Misuse of
    paternalism is of course a serious issue, and measures to prevent such misuse are
    needed: but refusal of treatment for the sake of marginal or missing autonomy
    is an even more serious one". I would suggest that similar considerations would
    apply, for example if an individual lacking capacity would benefit from partic-
    ipating in a health surveillance program. However, as I pointed out in the main
    text, *we* should not be making that decision, but rather it should be someone in
    a guardian role, on their behalf.
23. See also Laurie GT, Harmon SHE and Porter G. Mason and McCall Smith's
    Law and Medical Ethics. 2016, 10th edition. Oxford University Press, p. 460:
    "In some circumstances, it may be appropriate to take the basically paternalistic
    route to management and apply a 'best interests' test." This is in the context
    of treatment of mental illness, and they also point out that "it is important
    to reiterate that capacity is rarely an all-or-none affair; we should respect the
    decisions of individuals that they remain capable of making despite the presence
    of mental illness."
24. Zhou AY, Tamin J, Turner S and Menzies D. Severe learning disabilities and
    consent. Occupational Medicine, 2018, 68, 8, pp. 494–495. This provides a
    commentary for the situation in UK OH practice with regards to capacity and
    consent for those workers with severe learning disabilities.

Notes to Chap. 4

Confidentiality
Confidentiality and healthcare

1. Gillon R. Philosophical medical ethics. 1985. John Wiley & Sons. "The principle of medical confidentiality- that doctors must keep patients' secrets- is one of the most venerable moral obligations of medical ethics" (p. 106).
2. Case P. Confidence matters: The rise and fall of informational autonomy in medical law. Medical Law Review. 2003, 11, pp. 208–236. "The centrality of confidentiality to the therapeutic relationship is widely accepted, one of its functions being to facilitate trust between professions and their clients." (p. 209).
3. Kloss D. Occupational Health Law. 2010. Wiley-Blackwell, 5th edition. "The duty to keep secrets is enshrined in all codes of medical ethics." (p. 64).
4. General Medical Council. Confidentiality: Disclosing information for employment, insurance and similar purposes. 2017, para. 1, p. 10: "Trust is an essential part of the doctor-patient relationship and confidentiality is central to this. Patients may avoid seeking medical help, or may under-report symptoms, if they think their personal information will be disclosed by doctors without consent, or without the chance to have some control over the timing or amount of information shared."
5. For an elaboration of the justifications for an obligation of confidentiality, see Beauchamp TL and Childress JF. Principles of Biomedical Ethics. 2013. Cambridge University Press, 7th edition, pp. 319–320.

Confidentiality and OH practice

6. ICOH (2014). Medical confidentiality: "Individual medical data and the results of medical investigations must be recorded in confidential medical files which must be kept secured under the responsibility of the occupational health physician or the occupational health nurse. Access to medical files, their transmission and their release are governed by national laws or regulations on medical data where they exist and relevant national codes of ethics for health professionals and medical practitioners. The information contained in these files must only be used for occupational health purposes." (p. 25 para. 21).
7. See also, Westerholm P, Nilstun T, Ovretveit J (Eds.). Practical ethics in occupational health. Radcliffe Medical Press. 2004. In the context of work disability assessment in the Netherlands, the reasons for OH confidentiality being a "key principle" are given as: "First, if the patient is not able to divulge all necessary information, this could harm treatment. Second, autonomy of the patient would require prior consent before any such information is released. Third, the physician's loyalty is supposed to be with the patient in the first instance." (at p. 110). Although I agree with the reasons, I believe that these are subject to qualification and clarification, which I aim to do in this section (in the main text).

Privacy

8. See Laurie GT, Harmon SHE and Porter G. Mason and McCall Smith's Law and Medical Ethics. 2016, 10th edition. Oxford University Press, for a succinct and helpful explanation of the difference between privacy and confidentiality: "Privacy consists of two aspects: informational privacy and spatial privacy. Informational privacy is concerned with the control of personal information and with preventing access to that information by others. An invasion of informational privacy occurs when any unauthorized disclosure of information takes place. Confidentiality is a subset of this privacy interest and is breached when confidential information which is the subject of the relationship is released to parties outside the relationship without authorization. Informational privacy is wider than this in that it does not require a relationship to exist". (p. 241).

9. For an explanation of the justifications for a Right to Privacy, see Beauchamp TL and Childress JF. Principles of Biomedical Ethics. 2013. Cambridge University Press, 7th edition, pp. 313–314.

10. See also Laurie GT. Genetic privacy—a challenge to medico-legal norms. 2002. Cambridge University Press. He lists the reasons for protecting privacy as follows: "First, a state of physical separateness from others is necessary in order to allow personal relationships to begin and to grow…Second, a degree of separateness allows the individual personality to reflect on experiences and to learn from them…Third, it has been said that the modern psychological make-up of individuals is such that a degree of separateness is required to ensure that individuals retain a degree of mental stability…Fourth, tangible harm can come to an individual who is not granted a degree of privacy." (pp. 7–8). In terms of harm arising from invasion of one's informational privacy, he cites "information about one's personal condition, behavior or habits that others find distasteful can lead to individuals being ostracized by communities or becoming the object of violence and discrimination" (p. 8).

11. A right to privacy is protected for example in Article 8 of the European Convention on Human Rights www.echr.coe.int/Documents/Convention_ENG.pdf: "Everyone has the right to respect for his private and family life, his home and his correspondence". As previously mentioned in chapter 1, the UN Universal Declaration of Human Rights 1948, Article 12, also protects a right to privacy.

12. In Europe, Data Protection legislation is enacted through the General Data Protection Regulations (GDPR), https://www.eugdpr.org/

13. I have described a privacy paradigm based on the restricted access and limited control approach in Tamin J. What are "patient secrets" in occupational medicine practice? Privacy and confidentiality in "dual obligation doctor" situations. Medical Law International. 2015, pp. 1–30. https://doi.org/10.1177/0968533215587051, pp. 27–29.

Allowed disclosures

14. Singleton P, Lea N, Tapuria A and Kalra D. (Cambridge Health Informatics). General Medical Council: Public and Professional attitudes to privacy

of healthcare data, A Survey of the Literature. GMC, London, 2007. They provide empirical evidence of public uncertainty about medical confidentiality (at p. 27).

15. Kottow MH. Medical confidentiality: an intransigent and absolute obligation. Journal of Medical Ethics, 1986, 12, pp. 117–122. He argues that there should not be any allowed breaches of medical confidentiality, even in the public interest: "if physicians become known as confidence-violators, problem-ridden patients will try to lie, accommodate facts to their advantage or, if this does not work, avoid physicians altogether. Physicians would then be unable to give optimal advice or treatment to the detriment of both the reluctant patients and their threatened environment" (p. 120). Although Kottow was probably very aware of the political pressures in the Chile of the 1980s, I believe his view is worth noting even outside that context. It ought to make us think of how we justify disclosures, even with the very best of intentions, when we aim to gain public trust.

16. Warwick SJ. A vote for no confidence. Journal of Medical Ethics, 1989, 15, pp. 183–185. Warwick argues that the fact that breaches of confidentiality are allowed or even required would cause patient *mistrust* rather than trust, and on that basis that doctors should **not** accept information in confidence. She also describes the uncertainty around patients' expectations of what is to be kept secret, and for what reason, in the current "confidentiality" paradigm (p. 183).

17. See for example in the UK, General Medical Council. Confidentiality: Disclosing information for employment, insurance and similar purposes. 2017, p. 13: "Confidentiality is an important ethical and legal duty but it is not absolute. You may disclose personal information without breaching duties of confidentiality when any of the following circumstances applies:

   a. The patient consents, whether implicitly for the sake of their own care or for local clinical audit, or explicitly for other purposes (see paragraphs 13–15).
   b. The disclosure is of overall benefit to a patient who lacks the capacity to consent (see paragraphs 41–49).
   c. The disclosure is required by law (see paragraphs 17–19), or the disclosure is permitted or has been approved under a statutory process that sets aside the common law duty of confidentiality (see paragraphs 20–21).
   d. The disclosure can be justified in the public interest (see paragraphs 22–23)."

18. Beauchamp TL and Childress JF. Principles of Biomedical Ethics. 2013. Cambridge University Press, 7th edition, provides a risk assessment chart which can be helpful in understanding how to balance the conflicting ethical requirements of patient confidentiality and disclosing information to prevent harm to others (at p. 321).

How does this affect OH practice?

19. In the US case *Bratt* v. *IBM*, 392 Mass. 508 (1984), it was held that "In determining whether a physician's disclosure of medical information about an employee to his employer constitutes an actionable invasion of privacy under G. L. c. 214,

Section 1B, it is necessary to balance the degree of intrusion on the employee's privacy and the public interest in preserving the confidentiality of a physician-patient relationship against the employer's need for the information.".... "we conclude that when medical information is necessary reasonably to serve such a substantial and valid interest of the employer, it is not an invasion of privacy, under Section 1B, for a physician to disclose such information to the employer." The company doctor had disclosed information from a psychiatric assessment, that described Bratt as paranoid, to managers.

20. Commenting on the *Bratt* case, Beauchamp TL and Childress JF. (2013) at p. 319 state: "In our view, it is a reasonable conclusion that such information is not confidential by the standards of medical confidentiality relevant to this case and that Nugent (the IBM physician) was not bound by obligations of confidentiality in the same way a private physician would have been. Contracts calling for such limited disclosure are legitimate as long as employees are aware of, or should be aware of, provisions in the contract...Nevertheless, the company and the military, along with the physicians in each context, have a moral responsibility to ensure that employees and soldiers understand, at the outset, the conditions under which rules of confidentiality and protection of privacy do and do not apply."

21. UK courts have taken a similar approach to the US case of *Bratt*. In *Farnsworth v London Borough of Hammersmith & Fulham [2000] IRLR 691*, which was a pre-employment assessment case where Farnsworth claimed that the OH physician had breached her confidentiality in disclosing information to the managers, the courts (an Employment Appeal Tribunal) said: "A duty of confidence is one which prevents the holder of confidential information from using it or disclosing the information for purposes other than those for which it has been provided without the consent of the person to whom the duty of confidence is owed." Given that the purpose was a pre-employment assessment (for which she needed to obtain Farnsworth's consent), then the OH physician did not require *further* permission to disclose the results of her assessment to the relevant managers. She did not breach confidentiality in so doing.

22. For further pertinent comment, see Laurie GT, Harmon SHE and Porter G. Mason and McCall Smith's Law and Medical Ethics. 2016, 10th edition. Oxford University Press. At p 205: "A workplace doctor who is employed to carry out regular examinations on staff is bound by the terms of his or her contract to deliver information to the employer if this might have a bearing on the employer's business...It must now be stated explicitly before carrying out a pre-employment medical examination, or fitness to work, that the results of that examination may be communicated to the employer and the written consent of the examinee should be obtained in the light of that information." I agree with the authors. However, I believe that *"may* be communicated to the employer" (italics added) should in fact read "**will** be communicated to the employer", as the purpose of a pre-employment or fitness to work assessment is precisely to *advise* the employer of the result of this assessment.

23. For further commentary on confidentiality in OH, see Tamin J. What are "patient secrets" in occupational medicine practice? Privacy and confidentiality in "dual obligation doctor" situations. Medical Law International. 2015, pp. 1–30. https://doi.org/10.1177/0968533215587051.
24. For a succinct account of the tensions in OH practice around confidentiality, see Westerholm P, Nilstun T, Ovretveit J (Eds.). Practical ethics in occupational health. Radcliffe Medical Press. 2004, pp. 110–111. I will later address some of the issues the authors mention, in chapter 6 ("Report writing").

Notes to Chap. 5

Sickness absence
Introduction

1. I am indebted to Prof dr. Lode Godderis, Professor of Occupational, Environmental and Insurance Medicine at the Catholic University of Leuven, Belgium, for the following explanation: "a Belgian OH physician does not usually get involved with sickness absence, unless the worker contacts him. Under Belgian law, OH physicians are not allowed to make first contact with a worker while the latter off sick, except to establish whether the absence could be work-related. During the initial 2–4-week period, the worker could be assessed by a "cover doctor" paid for by the employer, in addition to the worker's own GP. If the worker remains off work beyond this initial period, he receives payments by an insurance scheme (also known as a 'mutual' or 'sickness fund') for up to a year at 60% of a limited wage rate. During that period, it is a sickness fund doctor that assesses the worker's fitness to resume work and the OH physicians have **no** role in this. The OH physician only sees a worker on his resuming work, to advise the employer on any required work adjustments. The sickness fund doctor and the OH physician are distinct roles carried out by different doctors, and neither performs the role of the other. In terms of their respective training schemes, the doctors follow separate courses (that is, either occupational or insurance medicine) and achieve different qualifications, although there are some modules that they both study, such as disability legislation." (personal communication).
2. For further insights into how the Belgian sickness absence system operates, see Du Bois M, Donceel P. Guiding low back claimants to work: a randomized controlled trial. Spine, 2012, 37:1425-31; and Du Bois M, Szpalski M, Donceel P. Patients at risk for long-term sick leave because of low back pain. Spine, 2009, 9:350-9.

Health, work and the disadvantaged

3. Dame Carol Black Report, Working for a healthier tomorrow, 2008. London: TSO; states that "The annual economic costs of sickness absence and workless-ness associated with working age ill-health are estimated to be over £100 billion." (at p. 10).

4. For further reading on ethical issues arising in sickness absence management, see Westerholm P, Nilstun T, Ovretveit J (Eds.). Practical ethics in occupational health. Radcliffe Medical Press. 2004, pp. 115–131. The situation in the Nether-lands is described, where following new legislation, employers had to continue to pay a worker for the first year of sickness absence, so they became more concerned about managing this. The authors comment that "the new legislation gives rise to many conflicts of interest. With regard to professional dilemmas, we observe that the well-being and the autonomy of employees, the financial inter-ests of employers and the professional role and position of occupational health professionals may all be involved." (at p. 115).

5. ICOH (2014): "On the basis of the principle of equity, occupational health professionals should assist workers in obtaining and maintaining employment notwithstanding their health deficiencies or their handicap." (para. 3, p. 11).

6. For a description of "vulnerable worker", see Rantanen J, Lehtinen S, Valenti A and Iavicoli S. Occupational health services for all—a global survey on OHS in selected countries of ICOH members. ICOH:2017. At p. 14:

Though the definitions of a vulnerable worker may vary depending on the context, the European, ILO and UN experts recognize three main groups of vulnerable workers:

1. *Economically and socially vulnerable workers*, including own account workers, unpaid family workers, young workers, unemployed workers, migrants and working poor, pre-carious workers, temporary agency workers, and informal sector workers. Their health and poverty situation is multifactorial and they need comprehensive social, health, and occupational health and safety programmes.

2. *Workers employed in jobs with high occupational safety and health risks:* in construction, mining, fishery, agriculture, and small-scale enterprises, and self-employed and informal sector and domestic workers. These workers need protective health and safety measures at their workplaces, particularly in the work environment.

3. *Workers vulnerable because of their health or psychophysiological situation:* workers with chronic medical conditions, and disabilities, as well as female workers, child and young adult workers, older workers, and workers vulnerable because of physiological or psychological factors. These workers require adjustments to their working conditions, work methods, work environment and work tasks to suit their work abilities and other capacities. Careful follow-up of their health at work is needed.

These different groups of vulnerable workers need different preventive, protective and pro-motional methods and specially adjusted services, which should be tailored according to their personal needs. Properly trained occupational health service personnel is in key position to provide such services.

7. Choi E. Health inequalities among Korean employees. Safety and Health at Work. 2017, 8, pp. 371–377. This study found "cumulative vulnerability caused

by the overlap in low social status, and this affects adverse work environments and poor health outcomes." (p. 377). This finding supports my suggestion in the main text that vulnerability of workers can be multi-dimensional, that is, those of lower social status (linked to lower income and poor educational achievement) are more likely to work in jobs that may adversely affect their health, and therefore their vulnerability is compounded.

8. WHO (Europe). Social Determinants of Health: The solid facts. 2nd edition, 2003. This publication provides us with some salient features of the social determinants of health, and some are particularly relevant to the contributions that OH could make in ameliorating these. For example: "Poverty, relative deprivation and social exclusion have a major impact on health and premature death" (p. 16); "Absolute poverty—a lack of the basic material necessities of life-continues to exist, even in some of the richest countries of Europe. The unemployed, many ethnic minority groups, guest workers, disabled people, refugees and homeless people are at particular risk of absolute poverty." (p. 16); but secure work could reverse this situation: "Job security increases health, wellbeing and job satisfaction. Higher rates of unemployment cause more illness and premature death." (p. 20). However, "because **very unsatisfactory or insecure jobs can be as harmful as unemployment**, merely having a job will not always protect physical and mental health: job quality is also important". (p. 20).

9. Choi's (2017) study (Note 7 above) based on data from over 27,000 employees in the Korean Working Condition Survey concluded that the "key social determinants of occupational health in Republic of Korea were precarious employment and manual labor occupations." (p. 377).

10. Waddell G and Burton AK. Is work good for your health and well-being? London, TSO:2006. This was a review of the evidence of the effect of work on health, and it concluded that **good** work is good for health.

11. Marmot M. Fair Society, Healthy Lives: Strategic Review of Health Inequalities in England post-2010. "The Marmot Re-view":2010. "Good work is characterised by a living wage, having control over work, in-work development, flexibility, protection from adverse working conditions, ill health prevention and stress management strategies and support for sick and disabled people that facilitates a return to work. Both the psychosocial and physical environments at work are critical." (p. 115).

12. See also Marmot M. Capabilities, Human Flourishing and the Health Gap, Journal of Human Development and Capabilities. 2017. 18:3, pp. 370–383 for valuable insights on how social fairness or unfairness strongly affects health.

13. For further commentary on vulnerable workers and OH, see Tamin J and Rajput-Ray M. 1.5 billion vulnerable workers and the role of OH professionals. ICOH Newsletter, December 2018, 16(3), pp. 24–27.

Disability

14. United Nations Convention on the Rights of Persons with Disabilities (UNCRPD). 2006. http://www.un.org/disabilities/documents/convention/convention_accessible_pdf.pdf: "Persons with disabilities include those who

have long-term physical, mental, intellectual or sensory impairments which in interaction with various barriers may hinder their full and effective participation in society on an equal basis with others." (Article 1, p. 3).

15. Mitra S. Disability, Health and Human Development. Palgrave Macmillan:2017. "Disability is associated with a higher likelihood of experiencing multidimensional poverty. These deprivations can be in terms of employment, health, education, material wellbeing, social participation or psychological wellbeing." (p. 93).

16. Sen A. The Idea of Justice. Penguin Books:2010. "The impairment of income-earning ability, which can be called the 'earning handicap' tends to be reinforced and much magnified by the 'conversion handicap': the difficulty in converting incomes and resources into good living, precisely because of disability." (p. 258).

17. Kuklys W. Amartya Sen's Capability Approach: Theoretical insights and Empirical Applications. Springer:2005. In her study of UK disabled households, Kuklys comments that "a disabled individual has a consumption opportunity set which is significantly reduced compared to a non-disabled individual. Our point estimates indicate that this reduction is of the order of 40%. It is important to reiterate that this reduction occurs despite the fact that many disabled individuals already receive compensation benefits and other allowances to help them with the additional cost." (p. 99).

18. Fevre R, Foster D, Jones M, and Wass V. Closing Disability Gaps at Work. Cardiff University:2016. This report was the result of in-depth analyses of data and empirical research in the UK into the situation of disabled workers. It makes for uncomfortable reading, especially in the worker's testimonies. For example, a nurse of 24 years' service who became a wheelchair user shared the following account of her experience: "My manager thought it was a huge joke to put his metal briefcase under the fax machine so I couldn't get my feet under. I couldn't see the buttons on it because it was at my eye level and I couldn't actually manage to do any faxing until I'd moved his briefcase out of the way." (p. 35). Such accounts of humiliation at work in this way may not come as a surprise to my fellow OH professional colleagues. I have had similar accounts from disabled workers and felt deeply ashamed that their colleagues and mangers could act in this manner. As OH professionals, we can empathize with a disabled worker treated like this, but we should also strive to make their colleagues and managers aware that such behaviour is not acceptable.

19. Fevre R. Why work is so problematic for people with disabilities and long-term health problems. Occupational Medicine. 2017, 67:593–595. Fever reports that in the UK, disabled employees are more likely to be in part-time jobs; to be paid less, to have fewer opportunities for training and development; and are more likely to have their employment rights infringed. They also experience difficulties during employment "which are not caused by their impairments or long-term health problems but can be traced to the behaviour of employers, managers and other employees" (p. 593). Of particular relevance to this chapter on sickness absence, he also comments that "any attempts by employers to

bear down on the costs of sickness absence may well have a disproportionate effect on disabled employees and contribute to the disability employment gap by causing them to leave their jobs." (p. 593).

Theories of justice

20. Rawls J. A theory of Justice. Harvard University Press:1977. (Revised edition). Rawls describes his conception of social justice as being based on two principles: "The first requires equality in the assignment of basic rights and duties, while the second holds that social and economic equalities of wealth and authority, are just only if they result in compensating benefits for everyone, and in particular for the least advantaged members of society." (p. 13).
21. Daniels N. Just Health- Meeting health needs fairly. Cambridge University Press:2008. "Examining the social determinants of health from the perspective of Rawls's theory is particularly appealing because justice as fairness is egalitarian in orientation and yet justifies certain inequalities, such as those in income and wealth, that contribute to health inequalities. In addition, my extension of Rawls links the protection of health to the protection of equality of opportunity, again setting up the potential for internal conflict." (p. 92).
22. Beauchamp TL and Childress JF. Principles of Biomedical Ethics. 2013. Cambridge University Press, 7th edition. The authors give a succinct account of the various theories of justice as follows (pp. 252–253): "Each theory articulates a general, notably abstract, material principle of distributive justice:

    i.   To each person according to rules and actions that maximise social utility. (*Utilitarian*).

    ii.   To each person a maximum of liberty and property resulting from the exercise of liberty rights and participation in fair free-market exchanges. (*Libertarian*).

    iii. To each person according to principles of fair distribution derived from conceptions of the good developed in moral communities. (*Communitarian*).

    iv. To each person an equal measure of liberty and equal access to the goods in life that every rational person values. (*Egalitarian*).

    v.   To each person the means necessary for the exercise of capabilities essential for a flourishing life. *(Capability)*.

    vi. To each person the means necessary for the realization of core dimensions of well-being. *(Well-being)*."

        Note: I have added the name of the relevant theory of justice (not included in the original text) in *italics* at the end of each sentence of this list for ease of understanding.

The capability approach

23. For those who are interested in reading more about the capability approach, I would recommend this very accessible and inspiring book: Sen A. The Idea of Justice. Penguin Books:2010. He describes the capability approach thus: "It

gives a central role to a person's *actual* ability to do different things that she values doing. The capability approach focuses on human lives, and not just on the resources that people have, in the form of owning—or having use of—objects of convenience that a person may possess. Income and wealth are often taken to be the main criteria of human success. By proposing a fundamental shift in the focus of attention from the *means* of living to the *actual opportunities* a person has, the capability approach aims at a fairly radical change in the standard evaluative approaches widely used in economics and social studies." (p. 253).

24. See also, Robeyns I. Wellbeing, Freedom and Social Justice: The capability approach re-examined. Open Book Publishers:2017. "The capability approach asks: *What are people really able to do and what kind of person are they able to be?* It asks what people can do and be (their capabilities) and what they are actually achieving in terms of beings and doings (their functioning's). Do the envisioned institutions, practices and policies focus on people's capabilities, that is, their opportunities to do what they value and be the kind of person they want to be?" (p. 9).

25. Nussbaum MC. Creating Capabilities: The Human Development Approach. The Belknap Press of Harvard University Press:2011. See particularly at pp. 32–34: "Considering the various areas of human life in which people move and act, this approach to social justice asks, what does a life worthy of human dignity require? At a bare minimum, an ample threshold level of the ten Central Capabilities is required. Given a widely shared understanding of the task of government (namely, that government has the job of making people able to pursue a dignified and minimally flourishing life), it follows that a decent political order must secure to all citizens at least a threshold of these ten Central Capabilities: 1. Life. 2. Bodily health. 3. Bodily integrity. 4. Senses, imagination, and thought. 5. Emotions. 6. Practical reason. 7. Affiliation. 8. Other species. 9. Play. 10. Control over one's environment (A) Political (B) Material."

    Note: Nussbaum does explain further each of these ten Central Capabilities, but I have not included her explanations here.

26. Rantanen J, Lehtinen S, Valenti A and Iavicoli S. Occupational health services for all- A global survey on OHS in selected countries of ICOH members. ICOH:2017. "The reported occupational health service coverage data were correlated with the UNDP Human Development Index. The HDI in high-OHS coverage countries is better than that in the low-coverage countries." (p. 56).

27. UNDP, at http://hdr.undp.org/en/content/human-development-index-hdi: "The HDI was created to emphasize that people and their capabilities should be the ultimate criteria for assessing the development of a country, not economic growth alone. The HDI can also be used to question national policy choices, asking how two countries with the same level of GNI per capita can end up with different human development outcomes. These contrasts can stimulate debate about government policy priorities. The Human Development Index (HDI) is a summary measure of average achievement in key dimensions of

human development: a long and healthy life, being knowledgeable and have a decent standard of living."

28. Sen A. Development as Freedom. Oxford University Press:1999. "The United Nations Development Programme (UNDP) has been publishing annual reports on "human development" that have thrown systematic light on the actual lives lived by people, especially the relatively deprived." (p. 73).

29. Van der Klink JJL, Bültmann U, Burdorf A, Schaufeli WB, Zijlstra FRH, Abma FI, Brouwer S, Van der Wilt GJ. Sustainable employability—definition, conceptualization, and implications: A perspective based on the capability approach. Scand J Work Environ Health. 2016, 42(1):71–79. "We propose a conceptual model of how resources, context, sustainable employability, and values might be related. This model is based on the concept of capability, as developed by Amartya Sen. Briefly, this model holds that an individual's sustainable employability is determined by how he or she succeeds in converting resources into capabilities, and subsequently into work functioning, in such a way that values such as security, recognition and meaning are met." (pp. 71–72). "An example of a valuable work functioning, important for many workers and one of the seven work values we identified in our research, is the opportunity to develop knowledge and skills. This value can be considered to be a (work) capability for a person if: (i) it is an important value for this person in his/her particular work situation; (ii) s/he is enabled by the work context (e.g., challenging tasks and an adequate HRM policy); and (iii) s/he is able to achieve it (e.g., the ability to learn). This combination of experiencing a value, being enabled, and being able, by means of both inputs and conversion factors, constitutes a (work) capability." (p. 74).

30. Abma FI, Brouwer S, de Vries HJ, Arends I, Robroek SJW, Cuijpers MPJ, van der Wilt GJ, Bültmann U, van der Klink JJL. The capability set for work: development and validation of a new questionnaire. Scand J Work Environ Health. 2016, 42(1):34–42. "The newly developed questionnaire to measure the capability set for work is unique because the items go beyond the valued aspects of work by incorporating whether a worker is able to achieve what he/she values in his/her work. The results show that the capability for work questionnaire can serve as a proxy measure of sustainable employability." (p. 34).

31. Abma FI, Bültmann U, Amick III BC, Arends I, Dorland HF, Flach PA, van der Klink JJL, van de Ven HA, Bjørner JB. The Work Role Functioning Questionnaire v2.0 Showed Consistent Factor Structure Across Six Working Samples. J Occup Rehabil. 2018, 28:465–474. A second version of the Work Role Functioning Questionnaire was validated, using over 2400 workers in 6 different working groups. The results indicate consistent structural validity across samples.

Unfair policies?

32. ICOH (2014): "The public or private institutions and organizations employing occupational health professionals should adopt a programme of organizational ethics that is aligned with the ethical principles of this Code." (p. 24, para. 19).

33. Iavicoli S, Valenti A, Gagliardi D, Rantanen J. Ethics and Occupational Health in the Contemporary World of Work. Int. J. Environ. Res. Public Health. 2018, 15, 1713; https://doi.org/10.3390/ijerph15081713. This important review of OH ethics endorses the ICOH Code statement at reference [32] above, and also reminds us of the important role of the ICOH Code itself: "The importance of the ICOH Code is reflected by the fact that national legislations (Argentina and Italy), international organizations (ILO, CIOMS, WHO), and other codes of ethics, post-graduate courses or treatises contain references to the subject. As far as the Italian national legal framework is concerned, pursuant to art. 39, c. 1 of Legislative Decree 81/08, "the activity of occupational physician is executed under the principles of occupational health and ICOH Code of Ethics". (At p. 8).

34. Iavicoli S et al. 2018. "We proposed an integrated approach to assessing the importance of all three types of ethics, personal (individual), professional and institutional, in resolving ethical conflicts." (p. 10). I mention this reference here, in relation to unfair policies, to note the importance of *institutional* ethics, as well as our own personal and professional ethics. The examples I have mentioned in this section, namely those of *Elsie* and of HCWs with an infective illness, can only really be resolved when the organizations concerned *also* aim to act ethically. I believe that in such situations our ethical behaviours alone cannot redress the injustices.

35. I would like to thank Professor Søren Holm, Professor of Bioethics at Manchester, Oslo and Aalborg Universities, for his conference presentation raising the issue of HCWs being penalized for being off work when they have influenza. His presentation at the 2013 ESPMH Conference was entitled "A Right to be Absent". He argued that if HCWs had "special obligations" (professional obligations, duty to do no harm), then Health Care Organizations also had special obligations, which would include not penalizing HCWs who have influenza "when they stay at home in good faith."

Conclusion

36. Nimmo S. Organizational justice and the psychological contract. Occupational Medicine. 2018, 68, pp. 83–85: "The evidence suggests that mental and physical health, sickness absence, job performance and job turnover are strongly correlated with organizational justice." (p. 84).

Notes to Chap. 6

Report writing
Pre-employment assessment reports

1. For a review of the evidence on pre-employment assessments, see Madan I and Williams S. A review of health screening of NHS staff. June 2010, London, TSO. They concluded that "only jobs where there are clear, explicit health criteria

should result in PEHS (pre-employment health screening). The screening should assess only the criteria identified as being essential for the job." (p. 30). Although their review was conducted for UK NHS staff, I believe that many of their findings and conclusions have wider applicability.

2. International Commission on Occupational Health (ICOH). International Code of Ethics for Occupational Health Professionals. 3rd edition, 2014: "The workers must be informed of the opportunity to challenge the conclusions concerning their fitness in relation to work that they feel contrary to their interest. An appeals procedure must be established in that respect." (p. 20, para. 9)

3. ICOH (2014): "The results of the examinations prescribed by national laws or regulations must only be conveyed to management in terms of fitness for the envisaged work or of limitations necessary from a medical point of view in the assignment of tasks or in the exposure to occupational hazards. In providing such information, the emphasis should be placed on proposals to adapt the tasks and working conditions to the abilities of the worker. General information on work fitness or in relation to health or the potential or probable health effects of work hazards, may be provided with the informed consent of the worker concerned, in so far as this is necessary to guarantee the protection of the worker's health." (p. 20, para. 10)

Management referral reports

4. The UK's regulatory approach to stress risk assessment (by the Health and Safety Executive-HSE) can be found at http://www.hse.gov.uk/stress/risk-assessment. htm. The Management Standards "help identify and manage six areas of work design which can affect stress levels-demand, control, support, relationships, role and change."

5. ICOH (2014): "The primary aim of occupational health practice is to safeguard and promote the health of workers, to promote a safe and healthy working environment, to protect the working capacity of workers and their access to employment". (p. 17, para. 1).

Ill-health retirement reports

6. Baron C and Poole J. Organizations and illness deception among employees, in Halligan PW, Bass C and Oakley DA (Eds.). Malingering and illness deception. Oxford University Press. 2003: "Malingering among employees is **rare** in our experience. Most patients present with an honest medical history, which is consistent with objective clinical findings and with the observations of third parties. **Most of our experience of illness deception has been encountered during the task of assessing financial awards associated with disability, usually in connection with applications for early retirement due to ill health or occupational injury awards.**" (p. 248, emphases added).

7. For an account of coercion and attempts at suppressing unfavourable OH physician IHR reports by applicants, see Ghani R. Complaints against healthcare workers. Occupational Health at Work, 2017, 14(2), pp. 13–18, at p. 15.

Self-referral reports

8. For notes on worker trust in OH, see chapter 2, notes 6–8.

Case conferences

9. Westerholm P, Nilstun T, Ovretveit J (Eds.). Practical ethics in occupational health. Radcliffe Medical Press. 2004: "The structure of consultation between occupational health physician, personnel manager and the other professionals involved often makes it difficult to comply strictly with requirements of confidentiality. Such consultation takes the form of the parties involved striving to solve a communal problem on the basis of equal involvement. The occupational health physician who appeals to confidentiality can easily be accused of not being committed to the solution of a troublesome sickness absence problem on the part of the company. From both a legal and ethical point of view, such a dilemma can only be resolved by requesting prior consent for discussing a patient's problem with third parties." (pp. 110–111).

10. See also Honkonen N, Liira J, Lamminpaa A and Liira H. Work ability meetings—a survey of Finnish occupational physicians. Occupational Medicine, 2018, 68, 8, pp. 551–554. This paper suggests that "Work ability meetings" (similar to the case conferences I have described) are a growing and popular intervention in Finnish OH practice. Work ability meetings "involve an employee, a manager and a representative of the occupational health service (OHS) meeting to discuss the employee's work ability or return to work." (p. 551). Given that the worker is present at these meetings, there may be fewer ethical problems with communication and disclosure of confidential worker information. However, one should still guard against overly intrusive questioning about sensitive medical matters by managers.

Notes to Chap. 7

Health Surveillance
Introduction

1. ICOH International Code of Ethics for Occupational Health Professionals (2014): "The aim of occupational health practice is to **protect and promote workers' health, to sustain and improve their working capacity and ability**, to contribute to the establishment and maintenance of a safe and healthy working environment for all..." (p. 11, emphases added).

Before the assessment

2. ICOH (2014): "Occupational health professionals must continuously strive to be familiar with the work and working environment as well as to develop their competence and to remain well informed in scientific and technical knowledge,

occupational hazards and the most efficient means to eliminate or to minimize the relevant risks. As the emphasis must be on primary prevention defined in terms of policies, design, choice of clean technologies, engineering control measures and adapting work organization and workplaces to workers, occupational health professionals must regularly and routinely, whenever possible, visit the workplaces and consult the workers and the management on the work that is performed." (p. 17).

3. ICOH (2014): "Biological tests and other investigations must be chosen for their validity and relevance for protection of the health of the worker concerned, with due regard to their sensitivity, their specificity and their predictive value. Occupational health professionals must not use screening tests or investigations which are not reliable or which do not have a sufficient predictive value in relation to the requirements of the work assignment." (p. 21).

4. Wilson JMG and Jungner G. Principles and practice of screening for disease. 1968, WHO: Geneva; From which come the following classic screening criteria:

   a. The condition sought should be an important health problem.
   b. There should be an accepted treatment for patients with recognized disease.
   c. Facilities for diagnosis and treatment should be available.
   d. There should be a recognizable latent or early symptomatic stage.
   e. There should be a suitable test or examination.
   f. The test should be acceptable to the population.
   g. The natural history of the condition, including development from latent to declared disease, should be adequately understood.
   h. There should be an agreed policy on whom to treat as patients.
   i. The cost of case-finding (including diagnosis and treatment of patients diagnosed) should be economically balanced in relation to possible expenditure on medical care as a whole.
   j. Case-finding should be a continuing process and not a "once and for all" project.

5. Andermann A, Blancquaert I, Beauchamp S, Dery V. Revisiting Wilson and Jungner in the genomic age: a review of screening criteria over the past 40 years. WHO Bulletin. 2008, Vol. 86, no. 4, pp. 241–320.

   Synthesis of emerging screening criteria proposed over the past 40 years:

   - The screening programme should respond to a recognized need.
   - The objectives of screening should be defined at the outset.
   - There should be a defined target population.
   - There should be scientific evidence of screening programme effectiveness.
   - The programme should integrate education, testing, clinical services and programme management.
   - There should be quality assurance, with mechanisms to minimize potential risks of screening.
   - The programme should ensure informed choice, confidentiality and respect for autonomy.

- The programme should promote equity and access to screening for the entire target population.
- Programme evaluation should be planned from the outset.
- The overall benefits of screening should outweigh the harm.

The assessment

6. ICOH (2014): "The surveillance must be carried out with the non-coerced informed consent of the workers. The potentially positive and negative consequences of participation in screening and health surveillance programmes should be discussed as part of the consent process. The health surveillance must be performed by an occupational health professional approved by a competent authority." (p. 20, para. 8).

7. An example of a competent authority approval for health surveillance is that of asbestos in the UK. The surveillance must be undertaken by an Appointed Doctor (by the Health and Safety Executive, HSE) under the Control of Asbestos at Work Regulations 2012.

8. Beauchamp TL and Childress JF. Principles of Biomedical Ethics. 2013. Cambridge University Press, 7th edition: "Coercion occurs if and only if one person intentionally uses a credible and severe threat of harm or force to control another." (p. 138).

9. We previously discussed a similar issue of possible coercion in chapter 6 (Pre-employment reports). My advice in the context of health surveillance is similar, that is, I believe that as OH professionals, we should ensure that the health surveillance program is as evidence-based, non-discriminatory and objective as possible. We should also ensure that the worker has a choice in accepting or refusing a particular course of action (in this case, a health surveillance assessment).

After the assessment

10. ICOH (2014): "The results of examinations, carried out within the framework of health surveillance must be explained to the worker concerned." (p. 20, para. 9).

11. ICOH (2014): "The results of the examinations prescribed by national laws or regulations must only be conveyed to management in terms of fitness for the envisaged work or of limitations necessary from a medical point of view in the assignment of tasks or in the exposure to occupational hazards. In providing such information, the emphasis should be placed on proposals to adapt the tasks and working conditions to the abilities of the worker." (p. 20, para. 10).

12. ICOH (2014): "Where the health condition of the worker and the nature of the tasks performed are such as to be likely to endanger the safety of others, the worker must be clearly informed of the situation. In the case of a particular hazardous situation, the management and, if so required by national regulations, the competent authority must also be informed of the measures necessary to safeguard other persons. In his advice, the occupational health professional must try to reconcile employment of the worker concerned with the safety or health of others that may be endangered." (pp. 20–21, para. 11).

13. ICOH (2014): "When there is no possibility of individual identification, information on aggregate health data on groups of workers may be disclosed to management and workers' representatives in the undertakings or to safety and health committees, where they exist, in order to help them in their duties to protect the health and safety of exposed groups of workers. Occupational injuries and work-related diseases must be reported to the competent authority according to national laws and regulations." (p. 25, para. 22). Although this statement states that "information on aggregate health data on groups of workers" *may* be disclosed, I believe that this should read "**must** be disclosed" instead. I think the intention of the ICOH code is likely to be the same, but the cautionary "*may*" is more in relation to the fact that individuals should not be identifiable, which I also agree is very important.

14. ICOH (2014): "Occupational health professionals must institute a programme of professional audit of their activities to ensure that appropriate standards have been set, that they are being met, that deficiencies, if any, are detected and corrected and that steps are taken to ensure continuous improvement of professional performance." (p. 26, para. 26). I am quoting this here in the context of health surveillance programs as they are a crucial OH activity which must be carried out to good professional standards. I will consider audit in our wider OH roles and functions in chapter 9.

Notes to Chap. 8

Vaccinations
Introduction

1. Nuffield Council on Bioethics. Public health: ethical issues. London. 2007: "Vaccinations involve treating a healthy person with a substance that is derived from (or similar to) a particular infectious disease agent. The purpose is to induce a response by the body that leads to enhanced immunity, and consequent protection, when exposed to the infectious agent in the future." (p. 53, para. 4.9).

Vaccinations and Public Health ethics

2. For an overview of vaccination ethics in population health discourses, see Nuffield Council on Bioethics (2007), pp. 53–58.

3. There is a further illuminating discussion of the "core controversial issue" of preventive vaccination in "Vaccination ethics" (chapter 8) in Dawson A (Ed.). Public Health Ethics: Key concepts and issues in policy and practice. Cambridge University Press:2011; pp. 143–153.

4. WHO, Measles, Mumps and Rubella (MMR), at http://www.who.int/biologicals/areas/vaccines/mmr/en/: "Combined live vaccine for measles, mumps and rubella (MMR) is used widely for the immunization of children in certain regions of the world because of its advantages over the individual vaccines."

5. Nuffield Council on Bioethics (2007): "MMR is given to both boys and girls, even though mumps is generally most serious for males and rubella is serious only for women during pregnancy. The rubella vaccine was previously given selectively only to girls, but this strategy was changed as pregnant women continued to contract the infection." (pp. 56–57, para. 4.18).

6. Nuffield Council on Bioethics (2007): "Free-riders are individuals who take more than their fair share of the benefits, or do not bear their fair share of the costs, of a resource or institution that is contributed to by many. Where population immunity exists and provides protection for those who refuse vaccination, it could be suggested that individuals who are not vaccinated are free-riders, as they do not share their fair burden, while nevertheless benefitting from population immunity. However, we find this suggestion unhelpful for understanding the complexities raised by vaccines. Although it is true that people pursuing such self-serving strategies would receive a personal benefit, not all who object to vaccinations or refuse them are motivated in this way. There are a range of other reasons for their objections: for example, people may not be convinced of the need for the vaccine, or may be concerned about its effects on themselves or their children." (p. 56, para. 4.17).

7. Nuffield Council on Bioethics (2007): "We identified two circumstances in which quasi-mandatory vaccination measures are more likely to be justified. First, for highly contagious and serious diseases, for example with characteristics similar to smallpox. Secondly, for disease eradication if the disease is serious and if eradication is within reach." (p. 60, para. 4.27).

8. Dawson A (Ed.). Public Health Ethics: Key concepts and issues in policy and practice. Cambridge University Press:2011: "Of course, 'compulsion' in the everyday sense implies the use of force or legal sanctions such as fines. However, related activities might count as 'indirect' compulsion and these can cover a range of cases from the requirement to have vaccinations before enrolment in school, to a presumption in favour of vaccination with little possibility to opt out and little attempt to offer the relevant information for an informed consent. Of course, direct compulsion will generally be an action of last resort." (p. 151).

9. Glover-Thomas N and Holm S. Compulsory vaccination, in Pioneering Healthcare Law. (Stanton C, Devaney S, Farrell AM and Mullock A, Eds.). Routledge, Oxon. 2016, pp. 31–42: "On balance, a wholly voluntary vaccination programme may no longer be tenable, and reflection is needed about whether coercion may offer the way forward." (p. 42).

Vaccinations and OH

10. I have previously considered more generally whether there are some lessons that we could learn from PH ethics. As we look after groups of workers as well as individual workers, I think it would be useful for us to consider the relevance of ethical values such as solidarity, which may need to be balanced against individual autonomy at times. I have included a transcript of the paper I presented at the Scottish SOM Spring 2016 Conference at Appendix 3 (Tamin J.

Occupational Health ethical confusion: Could Public Health ethics help? Sandy Elder Award 2014).

11. Hepatitis B vaccination in health care workers (HCWs) is summarized at https://www.who.int/occupational_health/activities/3hepatiti.pdf (Last accessed 20 November 2018).

12. The UK guidelines for occupational aspects of varicella zoster management, including vaccination, were published by the Royal College of Physicians (London) in 2010 and can be found at https://www.nhshealthatwork.co.uk/images/library/files/Clinical%20excellence/Varicella_zoster_guidelines_web_navigable.pdf (Last accessed 20 November 2018).

13. A summary of WHO recommendations for all HCW vaccinations can be found at http://www.who.int/immunization/policy/Immunization_routine_table4.pdf (Last accessed 1 December 2018).

Health care workers and flu vaccination

14. Greene MT, Fowler KE, Ratz D et al. Changes in influenza vaccination requirements for health care personnel in US hospitals. JAMA Netw Open 2018 Jun; 1: e180143. Available at https://doi.org/10.1001/jamanetworkopen.2018.0143 (last accessed 2 December 2018). This survey of 599 US hospitals in 2017 found that 61% of them had a mandatory flu vaccination program for HCWs.

15. Richardson S and Weaver K. Vaccinate-or-mask: Ethical duties and rights of health care providers in obtaining or refusing the influenza vaccination. Clinical Ethics. 2016, Vol 11(4), pp. 182–189. The authors maintain that a "vaccinate-or-mask" policy and mandatory HCW flu vaccination can be ethically justified by an analysis of the HCW's duty to protect the health and welfare of patients (especially from the deontological and utilitarian perspectives).

16. On the other hand, a Canadian arbitrator ruled against a group of Toronto hospitals arguing that the hospitals had failed to demonstrate that masks reduced flu infection and the "vaccinate or mask" policy aimed to compel staff to accept vaccination: see Dyer O. Flu vaccination: Toronto hospitals cannot implement staff "vaccinate or mask" policy, says ruling. BMJ 2018; 362 https://doi.org/10.1136/bmj.k3931 (published September 2018).

17. Tamin J. Mandatory flu vaccinations? Occupational Health at Work. 2016, 13(3), pp. 29–31. I have argued that, based on current evidence, it would *not* be morally right to make HCW flu vaccination mandatory for all groups of HCWs. The exception might be for staff in long-term elderly care settings, where the evidence is slightly stronger. However, even this evidence is weak (see below), so the evidential support for protection from flu vaccination remains sparse at this stage. A copy of this article is at Appendix 2.

18. Thomas RE, Jefferson T, Lasserson TJ. Influenza vaccination for healthcare workers who care for people aged 60 or older living in long-term care institutions. Cochrane Database of Systematic Reviews 2016; 6: CD005187. https://doi.org/10.1002/14651858. Available at https://www.cochrane.org/CD005187/ARI_influenza-vaccination-healthcare-workers-who-care-people-aged-60-or-older-living-long-term-care (last accessed 3 December 2018). The authors

conclude: "Offering influenza vaccination to healthcare workers who care for those aged 60 or over in LTCIs may have little or no effect on laboratory-proven influenza (low quality evidence)."

19. O'Reilly F, Dolan GP, Nguyen-Van-Tam J, Noone P. Practical prevention of nosocomial influenza transmission, 'a hierarchical control' issue. Occupational Medicine. 2015, 65, pp. 696–700.

Notes to Chap. 9

Conclusions
A framework for OH ethics?

1. Franco G. Ethical analysis of the decision-making process in occupational health practice. Med. Lav. 2005, 96, pp. 375–382. The author proposed a two-step approach to addressing ethical problems. The first step would be to identify the relevant ethical principles. The second step would be to identify the stakeholders. The preferred ethical outcome would then be chosen on the basis of ethical costs and benefits.

2. Westerholm P. Professional Ethics in Occupational Health- Western European Perspectives. Industrial Health, 2007, 45, pp. 19–25. The author takes a similar theoretical approach to Franco's paper above, but the tabular form it suggests is helpful. The ethical principles of autonomy, beneficence and justice are presented in a table where the persons involved or affected are considered (that is, the employees, the employer/management, the OH professional, and staff of the OH service).

3. Westerholm P, Nilstun T, Ovretveit J (Eds.). Practical ethics in occupational health. Radcliffe Medical Press. 2004. The same table as at note 3 above is presented as the model for ethical analysis (at p. 44). This model is then used throughout the book to analyse practical examples with good effect. I still commend this approach. However, I argue in the main text that this may not be sufficient in more complex and demanding OH ethics cases.

4. Iavicoli S, Valenti A, Gagliardi D, Rantanen J. Ethics and Occupational Health in the Contemporary World of Work. Int. J. Environ. Res. Public Health. 2018, 15, 1713; https://doi.org/10.3390/ijerph15081713: "The ethical choices are not only based on balanced risk and benefit for various stakeholders, but there are a number of deontological aspects as well that go beyond the mere benefit domains. There is still no systematic approach for analysing the true extent of these issues and their solutions."

Learning from experience: ethical reflection

5. International Commission on Occupational Health (ICOH). International Code of Ethics for Occupational Health Professionals. 3rd edition, 2014: "Occupational health professionals must institute a programme of professional audit of their

activities to ensure that appropriate standards have been set, that they are being met, that deficiencies, if any, are detected and corrected and that steps are taken to ensure continuous improvement of professional performance." (p. 26, para. 26). Also note that the preceding sentence urged OH professionals to obtain support from workers, employers and other stakeholders to implement "the **highest standards of ethics** in occupational health practice" (emphasis added).

The future?

6. Iavicoli S et al. (2018): "Over the past decades many new issues have come to the fore, reflecting changes in the world of work, fragmentation, economic difficulties, demographic shifts, new technologies and, more generally, the impact of globalization. The workforce itself is also diversifying, with and increasing participation of women, migrants and older workers."

7. Westerholm P et al. (2004). Chapter 1 entitled "A changing life at work: ethical ramifications", by Westerholm himself, gives a good overview of the topic. Although this book was published in 2004, much of what he said then remains valid today. This maybe reflects the fact that what we consider "new" or "changing" has been thought about and talked about for quite some time. Particular topics of interest in this chapter include "Working life change", "Globalisation", "Work and human rights" and "Corporate social accountability in working life", all of which remain highly relevant today.

8. Steel J, Luyten J and Godderis L. Occupational Health: The Global Evidence and Value. 2018, SOM & KU Leuven. Available at https://www.som. org.uk/sites/som.org.uk/files/Occupational_Health_the_Global_Value_and_ Evidence_April_2018.pdf . In the chapter entitled "Future value of occupational health": "One example is that the more health-aware enterprises today go beyond the minimum legislative requirements and bring **corporate social responsibility and sustainability** into practice. These two concepts express the commitment of enterprises to engage actively in the community in which it operates. This undertaking can take place on different levels—environmental, climate, (gender or other) equality, human rights, consumer protection, and also (occupational) health and safety. It reflects the fact that enterprises are intimately connected with their environment, with influence flowing in both directions. It also fits well with the vision that occupational health should focus on the broader well-being of workers: instead of a focus on physical health, mental and social aspects should be included when developing an occupational health strategy." (p. 26). I fully agree with the author's comments.

9. Iavicoli S et al. (2018). The authors comment that "The most important "next step" useful to resolve ethical challenges should include: (a) The development of a corpus of ethical principles that adequately consider the changing world of work, demographic shifts, new technologies and, more generally, the impact of globalization." I am in agreement with them. They further suggest increasing ethics education, closer collaboration and cooperation with others and developing ethics scenarios to learn from, all of which I also completely agree with.

10. London L, Tangwa G, Matchaba-Hove R, Mkhize N, Nwabueze R, Nyika A, Westerholm P. Ethics in occupational health: deliberations of an international workgroup addressing challenges in an African context. BMC Med Ethics. 2014, 15:48. https://doi.org/10.1186/1472-6939-15-48. Available at https://www.ncbi.nlm.nih.gov/pubmed/24957477. This paper provides an interesting account of the ICOH Ethical Code being reviewed in the African context. Amongst its many lessons, it notes that "particular cultural emphasis in traditional African societies on collective responsibilities within the community impacts directly on how consent should be sought in occupational health practice" and that " in the African context, the inseparability of workplace and community means that efforts to address workplace hazards demand that actions for occupational health extend beyond just the workplace". I provide this as an example of work that could (and in my view, should) be done in various cultural contexts given the effect of globalization on OH ethics. Each cultural context would then be an additional "module" within the OH ethics framework (see main text).

Epilogue

I started this book by recounting Elsie's story in the prologue.

You may have asked yourself, why? How does this relate to OH ethics? Indeed, one of the book reviewers commented "Is that ethics or just really poor practice, poor management and lack of respect for another human being?" Yes, it is all these. But to my mind it is also about our compassion for our patients and the sense of injustice we feel when they are unfairly treated. It is about recognizing that we can feel distressed and helpless, and that many of our moral decisions are made against this backdrop.

I wrote the preface to set the tone for this book. I wanted to let you know that I intended to discuss ethics in the "real world" of OH practice which can be sometimes difficult and even distressing for practitioners. I prefer to teach and learn through shared experiences, shared vulnerabilities and reflection rather than through a didactic approach.

During my medical career, patients have been my greatest teachers. I thank Elsie with all my heart.

© Springer Nature Switzerland AG 2020
J. Tamin, *Occupational Health Ethics*,
https://doi.org/10.1007/978-3-030-47283-2

Bibliography

1. Abma FI, Brouwer S, de Vries HJ, Arends I, Robroek SJW, Cuijpers MPJ, van der Wilt GJ, Bültmann U, van der Klink JJL (2016) The capability set for work: development and validation of a new questionnaire. Scand J Work Environ Health. 42(1):34–42
2. Abma FI, Bültmann U, Amick III BC, Arends I, Dorland HF, Flach PA, van der Klink JJL, van de Ven HA, Bjørner JB (2018) The work role functioning questionnaire v2.0 showed consistent factor structure across six working samples. J Occup Rehabil 28:465–474
3. Andermann A, Blancquaert I, Beauchamp S, Dery V (2008) Revisiting Wilson and Jungner in the genomic age: a review of screening criteria over the past 40 years. WHO Bull 86(4):241–320
4. Baron C and Poole J (2003) Organizations and illness deception among employees. In: Halligan PW, Bass C and Oakley DA (eds) Malingering and illness deception. Oxford University Press.
5. Bartlett P (1997) Doctors as fiduciaries: Equitable regulation of the doctor-patient relationship. Med Law Rev 5:193–224
6. Beauchamp TL (2010) Autonomy and consent. In: Miller FG and Wertheimer A (eds) The ethics of consent. Oxford University Press, pp 55–78
7. Beauchamp TL (2011) Informed consent: its history, meaning and present challenges. Camb Q Healthc Ethics 20:515–523
8. Beauchamp TL and Childress JF (2013) Principles of Biomedical Ethics, 7th edn. Cambridge University Press
9. Brazier M and Lobjoit M (1999) Fiduciary relationship: An ethical approach and a legal concept? In: Bennett R and Erin CA (eds) HIV and AIDS testing: screening and confidentiality. Oxford University Press, pp 179–199
10. Brody H (1987) The physician-patient relationship: models and criticisms. Theoretical Medicine 8. D. Reidel Publishing Company, pp 205–220
11. Case P (2003) Confidence matters: the rise and fall of informational autonomy in medical law. Med Law Rev 11:208–236
12. Choi E (2017) Health inequalities among Korean employees. Safety and Health at Work. 8:371–377
13. Dame Carol Black Report (2008) Working for a healthier tomorrow. London
14. Daniels N (2008) Just health-meeting health needs fairly. Cambridge University Press
15. Dawson A (ed) (2011) Public health ethics: key concepts and issues in policy and practice. Cambridge University Press
16. Du Bois M, Szpalski M, Donceel P (2009) Patients at risk for long-term sick leave because of low back pain. Spine 9:350–359
17. Du Bois M, Donceel P (2012) Guiding low back claimants to work: a randomized controlled trial. Spine 37:1425–1431
18. Dworkin G (1988) The theory and practice of autonomy. Cambridge University Press
19. Dworkin R (2013) Taking rights seriously. Bloomsbury Academic

20. Dyer O (2018) Flu vaccination: Toronto hospitals cannot implement staff "vaccinate or mask" policy, says ruling. BMJ 362. https://doi.org/10.1136/bmj.k3931 (published September 2018)
21. European Convention on Human Rights www.echr.coe.int/Documents/Convention_ENG.pdf
22. Faculty of Occupational Medicine (2006) Guidance on ethics for occupational physicians, 6th edn. Faculty of Occupational Medicine of the Royal College of Physicians, London
23. Faculty of Occupational Medicine (2012) Ethics Guidance for Occupational Health Practice, 7th edn. Faculty of Occupational Medicine of the Royal College of Physicians, London
24. Fevre R, Foster D, Jones M, Wass V (2016) Closing Disability Gaps at Work. Cardiff University
25. Fevre R (2017) Why work is so problematic for people with disabilities and long-term health problems. Occup Med 67:593–595
26. Franco G (2005) Ethical analysis of the decision-making process in occupational health practice. Med Lav 96:375–382
27. French Code de Déontologie Médicale (Avril 2017)
28. General Medical Council (2017) Confidentiality: Disclosing information for employment, insurance and similar purposes
29. Ghani R (2017) Complaints against healthcare workers. Occup Health at Work 14(2):13–18
30. Gillon R (1985) Philosophical medical ethics. Wiley, Chichester
31. Glover-Thomas N and Holm S (2016) Compulsory vaccination. In: Stanton C, Devaney S, Farrell AM, Mullock A (eds) Pioneering healthcare law. Routledge, Oxon, pp 31–42
32. Greene MT, Fowler KE, Ratz D et al (2018) Changes in influenza vaccination requirements for health care personnel in US hospitals. JAMA Netw Open:e180143. https://doi.org/10.1001/jamanetworkopen.2018.0143
33. Honkonen N, Liira J, Lamminpaa A, Liira H (2018) Work ability meetings—a survey of Finnish occupational physicians. Occup Med 68(8):551–554
34. Iavicoli S, Valenti A, Gagliardi D, Rantanen J (2018) Ethics and Occupational Health in the Contemporary World of Work. Int J Environ Res Public Health 15:1713. https://doi.org/10.3390/ijerph15081713
35. International Commission on Occupational Health (ICOH) (2014) International code of ethics for occupational health professionals, 3rd edn
36. Kennedy I (1996) The fiduciary relationship and its application to doctors and patients. In: Birks P (ed) Wrongs and remedies in the twenty-first century. Oxford University Press, pp 111–140
37. Kloss D (2010) Occupational health law, 5th edn. Wiley-Blackwell
38. Kottow MH (1986) Medical confidentiality: an intransigent and absolute obligation. J Med Ethics 12:117–122
39. Kuhse H, Singer P (eds) (2012) A companion to bioethics, 2nd edn. Wiley-Blackwell
40. Kuklys W (2005) Amartya Sen's capability approach: theoretical insights and empirical applications. Springer
41. Laurie GT (2002) Genetic privacy—a challenge to medico-legal norms. Cambridge University Press
42. Laurie GT, Harmon SHE, Porter G (2016) Mason and McCall Smith's law and medical ethics, 10th edn. Oxford University Press
43. London L, Tangwa G, Matchaba-Hove R, Mkhize N, Nwabueze R, Nyika A, Westerholm P. Ethics in occupational health: deliberations of an international workgroup addressing challenges in an African context. BMC Med Ethics. 2014, 15:48. https://doi.org/10.1186/1472-6939-15-48, https://www.ncbi.nlm.nih.gov/pubmed/24957477
44. Madan I, Williams S (2010) A review of health screening of NHS staff. TSO, London
45. Manson NC, O'Neill O (2007) Rethinking informed consent in bioethics. Cambridge University Press
46. Marmot M. Fair Society, Healthy Lives: Strategic Review of Health Inequalities in England post-2010. "The Marmot Review":2010
47. Marmot M (2017) Capabilities, human flourishing and the health gap. J Hum Dev Capab 18(3):370–383

48. Martimo KP, Antti-Poika M, Leinof T, Rossit K (1998) Ethical issues among Finnish occupational physicians and nurses. Occup Med 48:375–380
49. Mitra S (2017) Disability, Health and Human Development. Palgrave Macmillan:
50. Nimmo S (2018) Organizational justice and the psychological contract. Occup Med 68:83–85
51. Nuffield Council on Bioethics (2007) Public health: ethical issues. London
52. Nuremberg Code 1947 https://history.nih.gov/research/downloads/nuremberg.pdf
53. Nussbaum MC (2011) Creating capabilities: the human development approach. The Belknap Press of Harvard University Press
54. O'Neill O (2002) A question of trust. Cambridge University Press
55. O'Neill O (2002) Autonomy and trust in bioethics. Cambridge University Press
56. O'Reilly F, Dolan GP, Nguyen-Van-Tam J, Noone P (2015) Practical prevention of nosocomial influenza transmission, 'a hierarchical control' issue. Occup Med 65:696–700
57. Pellegrino ED, Thomasma DC (1987) The Conflict between Autonomy and Beneficence in Medical Ethics: Proposal for a Resolution. Journal of Contemporary Health Law and Policy. 3(1):23–46
58. Plomp HN (1992) Workers' attitude toward the occupational physician. J Occup Med 34(9):893–901
59. Plomp HN, Ballast N (2010) Trust and vulnerability in doctor-patient relations in occupational health. Occup Med 60:261–269
60. Prainsac B, Buyx A (2011) Solidarity: reflections on an emerging concept in bioethics. A report commissioned by the Nuffield Council on Bioethics. ISBN: 978-1-904384-25-0
61. Rantanen J, Lehtinen S, Valenti A, Iavicoli S (2017) Occupational health services for all—a global survey on OHS in selected countries of ICOH members. ICOH. ISBN 978-889-434-692-3(pdf)
62. Rawls J (1977) A theory of justice, (revised edition). Harvard University Press
63. Richardson S, Weaver K (2016) Vaccinate-or-mask: Ethical duties and rights of health care providers in obtaining or refusing the influenza vaccination. Clin Ethics 11(4):182–189
64. Robeyns I (2017) Wellbeing, freedom and social justice: the capability approach re-examined. Open Book Publishers
65. Royal College of Physicians (2010) Varicella zoster virus: occupational aspects of management. https://www.nhshealthatwork.co.uk/images/library/files/Clinical%20excellence/Varicella_zoster_guidelines_web_navigable.pdf
66. Sen A (1999). Development as freedom. Oxford University Press
67. Sen A (2010) The idea of justice. Penguin Books
68. Sieghart P (1982) Professional ethics—for whose benefit? J Med Ethics:25–32
69. Singer P (ed) (1993) A companion to ethics. Blackwell
70. Singleton P, Lea N, Tapuria A, Kalra D, (Cambridge Health Informatics) (2007) General medical council: public and professional attitudes to privacy of healthcare data, A survey of the literature. GMC, London
71. Stanley JM (1989) The Appleton Consensus: suggested international guidelines for decisions to forego medical treatment. J Med Ethics 15:129–136
72. Steel J, Luyten J, Godderis L (2018) Occupational health: the global evidence and value, SOM & KU Leuven. https://www.som.org.uk/sites/som.org.uk/files/Occupational_Health_the_Global_Value_and_Evidence_April_2018.pdf
73. Stilz R, Madan I (2014) Worker expectations of occupational health consultations. Occup Med 64:177–180
74. Tamin J (2014) Can informed consent apply to information disclosure? Moral and practical implications. Clin Ethics 9(1):1–9
75. Tamin J (2014) Ethics guidance for occupational health practice: a commentary. Clin Ethics 9(2–3):61–62
76. Tamin J (2016) Mandatory flu vaccinations? Occup Health at Work 13(3):29–31
77. Tamin J (2013) Models of occupational medicine practice: an approach to understanding moral conflict in "dual obligation" doctors. Med Healthc Philos 16(3):499–506

78. Tamin J (2014) Occupational health ethical confusion: could public health ethics help? Sandy Elder Award, presented to the Scottish SOM Spring 2016 conference on the 28th April 2016. A transcript of this oral presentation is at Appendix 3
79. Tamin J (2015) What are "patient secrets" in occupational medicine practice? Privacy and confidentiality in "dual obligation doctor" situations. Med Law Int:1–30
80. Tamin J and Rajput-Ray M. 1.5 billion vulnerable workers and the role of OH professionals. ICOH Newsletter, December 2018, 16(3), pp 24-27
81. Tauber AI (2005) Patient autonomy and the ethics of responsibility. MIT Press
82. Thomas RE, Jefferson T, Lasserson TJ (2016) Influenza vaccination for healthcare workers who care for people aged 60 or older living in long-term care institutions. Cochrane Database Syst Rev 6:CD005187. https://doi.org/10.1002/14651858
83. United Nations Convention on the Rights of Persons with Disabilities (UNCRPD) (2006) http://www.un.org/disabilities/documents/convention/convention_accessible_pdf.pdf
84. UNDP (for UN Human Development Reports), at http://hdr.undp.org/en/content/human-development-index-hdi
85. United Nations (1948) Universal declaration of human rights. http://www.un.org/en/universal-declaration-human-rights/
86. Van der Klink JJL, Bültmann U, Burdorf A, Schaufeli WB, Zijlstra FRH, Abma FI, Brouwer S, Van der Wilt GJ (2016) Sustainable employability—definition, conceptualization, and implications: a perspective based on the capability approach. Scand J Work Environ Health 42(1):71–79
87. Waddell G, Burton AK (2006) Is work good for your health and well-being?. TSO, London
88. Warwick SJ (1989) A vote for no confidence. J Med Ethics 15:183–185
89. Westerholm P (2009) Codes of ethics—are they important? Ethical dilemmas and challenges in occupational health. CME 27(11):492–494
90. Westerholm P (2007) Professional ethics in occupational health—Western European perspectives. Ind Health 45:19–25
91. Westerholm P, Nilstun T, Ovretveit J (eds) (2004) Practical ethics in occupational health. Radcliffe Medical Press
92. WHO (Europe) (2003) Social determinants of health: the solid facts, 2nd edn
93. WHO, Measles, Mumps and Rubella (MMR). http://www.who.int/biologicals/areas/vaccines/mmr/en/
94. Wilson JMG, Jungner G (1968) Principles and practice of screening for disease. WHO, Geneva
95. Zhou AY, Tamin J, Turner S, Menzies D (2018) Severe learning disabilities and consent. Occup Med 68(8):494–495

Printed in the United States
by Baker & Taylor Publisher Services